What O

Breaking *the*
COVER GIRL MASK

God Bless —

Kimberly

Breaking the COVER GIRL MASK

Toss Out Toxic Thoughts

KIMBERLY DAVIDSON

TATE PUBLISHING & *Enterprises*

Published by Tate Publishing & Enterprises, LLC
127 E. Trade Center Terrace | Mustang, Oklahoma 73064 USA
1.888.361.9473 | www.tatepublishing.com

Tate Publishing is committed to excellence in the publishing industry. The company reflects the philosophy established by the founders, based on Psalm 68:11,
"The Lord gave the word and great was the company of those who published it."

Book design copyright © 2009 by Tate Publishing, LLC. All rights reserved.
Cover design by Amber Gulilat
Interior design by Jeff Fisher

Published in the United States of America

ISBN: 978-1-60799-847-1
1. Religion, Christian Life, Women's Issues
2. Self-Help, Personal Growth, Self-Esteem
09.09.01

Table of Contents

There is No Freedom
without a Change of Mind

If your mind was a movie screen for everyone to view, what would they see? Would your screenplay be rated G, R, or NC-17? The Apostle Paul confessed, "I do not understand what I do. For what I want to do, I do not do, but what I hate I do. I have the desire to carry out good but cannot carry it out" (Rom. 7:15; 18).

Ever feel this way? Maybe everyday! Philosopher and physician, Aristotle said, "We are what we repeatedly do."[1] If we want to understand why we do what we don't want to do, why we think and act negatively, then we must come to the realization we do not understand ourselves as well as we think we do.

Today, as never before, millions of Christian women, of all ages, are struggling in emotional and physical prisons. Depression, physical illness, emotional disorders, the trauma of abuse, and addiction create harmful thoughts literally embedded in their minds.

Unaware they have hidden brokenness, pain, and repressed memories, their relationships with others and with God are compromised. Living a life they cannot sustain and desperate for relief, they spend millions of dollars on mental health specialists, therapies, prescription medications and vitamin supplements.

People are searching as never before for direction and answers. Many women feel they will never be able to break free from the toxic thoughts that bind them. It can indeed be very difficult to change what we don't understand. But there is hope!

Do you *genuinely* desire to change and grow? Then, ask yourself what lies and wounds you hide? What accusations do you wear as your identity? What temptations are you continually enslaved to? You can break free from these kinds of toxic thoughts and emotions that bind you by implementing R.E.S.I.S.T. Experience true and powerful mind change, restoring the mind and nature Christ died to give you!

When school was let out for the day, either Mom or our babysitter, Annie, would meet my brother, age seven, and me, age ten, by the school playground, with the four-year-old in tote. Most days we'd go on to do something fun for a couple hours, like go to the park or a museum. Some days we were allowed to spend our allowances at Mrs. Seddon's candy shop.

On this particular day, Annie announced, "We're going straight home. Sorry, no fun stops today." Shocked, I asked why. She wouldn't give me an answer.

The next day she proclaimed the same thing, "We're going home."

"What! Two days in a row? Not fair. Why?" I cried. I still got no explanation. All she said was we weren't being punished, which surprised me.

"You can play in the yard." *Well, that's a real treat. Our yard is the size of postage stamp!*

The same thing happened the next day ... and the next. I got really mad. "None of my other friends have to go home after school!" I'm really thinking, *You are cruel and mean. I am being punished!*

This went on for almost two weeks. I was on the verge of a tantrum and Annie sensed it. She broke her code of silence. "I didn't want to tell you this because I didn't want to scare you. But you're being such a brat, I have no choice."

Scare me? What was going to come out next?

"They found a girl's naked body in a dumpster behind the library (which was two blocks away). They think it's connected to the other two neighborhood murders. Now do you understand why we are coming straight home? It's for our protection."

Now I understood. My crabapple attitude disappeared immediately. I was scared but now I wanted details. "How old was she? When and how was she abducted? Did she know the murderer? Tell me! Tell me!"

The more I could learn about this awful incident, the more I might avoid the same kind of horrible death. If you understand something, you can begin to control it instead of letting it control you. A wise woman once said, "I am never afraid of what I know."

In order for us to change lifelong patterns, we have to understand ourselves better. And who better to show us than the Almighty God, the one who created us and knows all our ways (Ps. 139:1–16). Knowledge changes everything!

Proverbs 2:10 says, "Wisdom will enter your heart and knowledge will be pleasant to your soul." Paul said, "Put on the new self, which is being renewed in knowledge in the image of its Creator" (Col. 3:10). God wants to re-make us into the image of his Son! How does that renewal come about? Through knowledge.

We are created in the image of God (Gen. 1:26–27). This involves our personality—intellect, emotion and will; and our spirituality. When man first sinned this image was ruined (Gen. 3). But through the work of Jesus Christ we can be transformed into God's image! This doesn't mean we become God, but as his creation we can mirror his image. First, we must renew our minds because our minds affects our whole being (Eph. 4:22–24).

At this very moment we are changing. We're aging! To most women that represents negative change. It is something we have no control over. What we do have control over is the desire and ability to change our mind (and how we react to aging).

We cannot live the life God intended, a life of freedom and joy, without a change of mind. As we grow in the knowledge of the Word of God we begin to make better choices, bear his glorious image (2 Cor. 3:18) as he starts the transformation process of renewing our minds (Rom. 12:2).

Have you ever walked around with food in your teeth? Until

you look into the mirror, you won't pluck that food out. God's Word is our mirror. When we look into it, it will show us what is missing, where we've gone wrong and instruct us how to fix it. It is truth, and it sets our minds free from toxic thinking. But first, spiritual growth requires the acknowledgement of our own need to grow.

Let's do an attitude check. If someone were to follow you around this week, how would they describe you?

1. Gracious or cranky?

2. Complimentary or critical?

3. Encouraging or bitter?

Our attitudes are important to health and success in life. Our lives affect those we have contact with, either positively or negatively. Because emotions and behaviors involve a complex interplay between the heart, the mind, and the body, it benefits us to know how our mind is influenced and how our brain works.

Your body believes every word you say! We do not merely experience anger in our minds, we feel it biologically in our body—our muscles tense and stomachs ache. Understanding ourselves, and other people, is critical to mind change and our overall growth. If we were to look at our brain, we may see a dark abscess caused by the stronghold of anger. The same is true for envy, anxiety, lust, fear, depression, and other emotions.

The Bible says, "A heart at peace gives life to the body, but envy rots the bones" (Prov. 14:30). There is a direct correlation between pessimistic, toxic thinking and illness. If we do not have a change of mind, we can actually make ourselves sick! Our body truly speaks our mind.

Even as a Christian, my mind continued to create negative thoughts, which translated into bad feelings and behaviors. Not only was my mind and heart tormented, but so was my physical body. I was diagnosed with lupus, gastritis, and shingles. No question, what you think influences your biological body. Toxic thinking can manifest itself in bodily symptoms such as cancer, diabetes, allergies, to name a few.[2]

Research confirms some of our behaviors actually prevent us from being our best selves. The reasons may be varied, from psychological or biological causes to spiritual warfare, or a combination. We know our brain speaks to our body and vice versa. There is an ongoing symphony of chemicals playing through your body twenty-four hours a day. Our way of thinking affects the functioning of that whole electrical-chemical cycle. When the cycle is upset, all sorts of illnesses and injuries can result, impairing our ability to decipher truth and live a fulfilling life.

Finding the root cause does not excuse bad behavior or lessen the need to seek spiritual or therapeutic help. Rather, it allows us to better understand why we do what we do so we might choose better alternatives.

The reason we have conflict is lack of information and indifference, "My people are destroyed from lack of knowledge" (Hos. 4:6). Knowledge is the investigation of the truth. It is important to understand how our past influences the present, which is part one of this book—the first leg of the journey. Then we move into part two—evaluate the present. Taking the principles and tools presented, we will begin refocusing the present and future (part three). Our final leg is a transformed mind. It is about being the best that we can be!

⁓

Getting the Most Out of this Experience

No doubt you picked up this book because you want a different future. I wish I could give you a few steps to instantly set your thinking back on God's track, but I can't. I do want to encourage and help you quicken the pace and learn the how. But no one else can do this for you.

This is a journey of self-discovery and examination. The Bible consistently teaches we are to evaluate ourselves honestly before God and others. God intends that we live in his image, as an exact likeness, having a high sense of self-esteem. We shouldn't be using our own standards of measurement to find out what's wrong with everybody else, but find out where we're missing the mark.

Digging deep and expressing our emotions is an important step to conquering toxic thoughts. Seeking the Holy Spirit's revelation of truth about ourselves can greatly increase our awareness of internal strengths, areas needing further growth, hidden pain and unresolved conflict. Practicing openness before the Lord can create greater vulnerability in our relationships.

My objective is for you to better understand your personality and put into practice mind change by discovering the connection between the *spiritual*—the light and the dark side of spiritual conflict; the *biological*—our brains and bodies; and the *psychological*—our minds and personalities: past, present, and future.

This book is designed to be done either as a small group or on your own. Each chapter contains a number of subheadings breaking the text up and concludes with a *Reflect* question to move the R.E.S.I.S.T. process forward. Keeping an inexpensive notebook or journal to answer the questions will help you remember and embrace action. If you do this on your own, set a goal each day of how many sections you want to complete.

As you reflect on each question, pray that God will provide you courage and insight to honestly answer. I challenge you to really evaluate, question, and think about what you read. Ask God to show you who you really are. Examine your own level of thinking. Dig for in-dept explanations. Take the time to look up the verses that are referenced. When you do, you are ingesting the living Word of God.

Everything God commands is for our good and enhances brain function and positive thinking. His Word is like a doctor's prescription, meant to make us well and happy (see Deut. 6:24; 10:12–13). You will soon discover who you truly are: a significant and secure woman who cannot be enslaved; someone who has the potential to be a loving, giving, and confident.

You will be asked to look up and mediate on Scripture verses. Meditation is often misunderstood. Eastern religion relies on emptying the mind of conscious thought. Christian meditation is filling the mind with knowledge of God, which is the lifelong process of remembering and musing over the Bible's teachings and promises, and then asking God how you should change. Our significance does not come from our own wisdom, might, or riches, but from knowing and understanding God (Jer. 9:23–24).

For us, true and powerful mind change comes as we evaluate, single out, and compare our thoughts to God's thoughts. Then we are in a position to make choices based on clear and concise biblical reasoning. It begins with a genuine desire and sincerity to see what is wrong with our thinking. For example, I'm thinking, *Preserve the face and body!* God's thinking, *I love her so much. I want to save her soul.*

Meet God in these pages. Spiritual growth is all about increasing relational closeness to Christ and is a learned behavior. Any one of us can cultivate it. God gives us twenty-fours hours a day, and we must make a commitment to give him an adequate amount of time. Seek God as David did. "Examine my heart and my mind for your love is ever before me. I walk continually in your truth" (Ps. 26:2–3).

I pastor women of all ages in emotional and transitional pain. I am a researcher who mines information. And I spent over twenty years working in the health sciences field. I have walked this walk…and continue to do so. Tiger Woods once said, "There's always stuff to work on. You're never there."[3]

Counselors and physicians do a great job of identifying emotional and physical issues and then prescribing solutions. As your spiritual guide, I want to help you become more skillful in the use of God's Word as a biblical foundation to meet your daily challenges.

You will be given proven techniques you can apply immediately to help optimize heart and mind, even brain, function. You will not only understand yourself better, but you'll understand why other people do what they do. *You can do this!* "For nothing is impossible with God" (Luke 1:37). Whatever your mind can conceive and believe, it can achieve, but there are certain conflict zones we must learn to resist.

I have dubbed this biblical process R.E.S.I.S.T.

- *Recognize* everyday you are in spiritual battle with the world, with yourself, and with an adversary. Recognize God's desire is to mold you into a woman that reflects Jesus in character, attitude, thought, and action.

- *Embrace* your God-designed personality and your birthright. Embrace the truth. You will never be more like Christ than when you are immersed in, and living out, biblical truth.

- *Submit* your thoughts to Christ. This means consciously handing over anxiety, worry, pain, and bitterness. He stands prepared to take your load and b*reak the chains of thought-bondage* if you let him.

- I*dentify & interrogate* the negative things and lies you say to yourself, thereby enabling yourself to replace distortions with truth.

- S*et your mind and heart on God,* thereby washing yourself of the will to run your own life.

- T*hank and praise God.* Through Jesus, continually offer God a sacrifice of praise (Heb. 13:15). He not only saved you from the clutches of sin, but he is also working to reconcile your inner conflicts, heal your brokenness, and change your entire life.

R.E.S.I.S.T. is not a step-by-step process, but an integrated lifestyle change. Take a look inside. See yourself as you really are! Jesus was angry with the Pharisees for looking at only the outside of their lives (Matt. 23:26). Cleaning up our insides is essential if we want to develop an intimate relationship with our Father.

We each face a dilemma the moment we say yes to Christianity:

1. Live in thought-bondage and allow our negative emotions to control us. Or,

2. Stay stagnant—spiritually, emotionally and relationally. Or,

3. Confront and conquer toxic thoughts and emotions, jump starting the maturation process of thinking and acting more like Jesus.

Socrates said the unexamined life is not worth living. Through prayer and self-examination, we can learn to submit our struggles because they are impossible to conquer in our own strength. Do you have an attitude of willingness to expose and examine your flaws? Yes! Let's go!

Strongholds, Mindholds

Has anyone ever said to you or insinuated, "You're so stupid," or "You'll never be able to do that," or "Don't you wish you were as pretty are her?" Perhaps you struggle with the shame of abuse or the anguish of battling depression. Over time, these negative comments or feelings usually become strongholds.

A stronghold is something that has a strong hold or powerful influence on a person. It is a mindset that is resistant to change. Synonyms are stranglehold, vice-like iron grip, cancer, and infection. It is a deeply entrenched pattern of thought, ideology, value, or behavior burnt into our minds through negative repetition.

I call these mental strongholds or habits, *mindholds*—harmful thoughts and emotions literally embedded in our minds. Mindholds temporarily make us feel good by filling that hole in our hearts. But, they can also be God's way of telling us we have some serious things to deal with.

The most common strongholds are fear, people-pleasing, low self-esteem, anger and unforgiveness, doubt, unbelief in God's character, perfectionism and bad habits. Over time, our habits and thoughts shape who we are. As we nurture them, we choose to bend our will until we no longer choose a different route, becoming a slave to that toxic thought or habit.

"My mom is addicted to chocolate, and so I am. I can't change. It's in my genes! I'll always be a chocoholic!" is a stronghold (sorry, ladies!). Like a slave, we submit ourselves to its wicked demands. It may even end up destroying us.

Mindholds (or strongholds) are also visible to the eye in a brain scan. Learning specialist, Dr. Caroline Leaf, author of *Who Switched Off My Brain?* states a stronghold literally looks like a cancer or abscess. For example, unforgiveness locks toxins in the body, which results in a heavy, dark memory. On the other hand, research shows an enriched environment of thinking positive, healthy thoughts can lead to significant structural changes in the brain's cortex.

Brain imaging illustrates that positive thoughts look like beautiful, lush, and healthy green trees. Whereas negative thoughts look like ugly, mangled, snarling thorn bushes.

Dr. Leaf asserts toxic thoughts build toxic memories. They upset the chemical feedback loops in your brain by putting your body in a harmful state. Your brain grows heavy with thick memories that release a toxic load, interfering with function.[4] She says that if you have been repeatedly verbally or sexually abused as a child, all the thoughts associated with those experiences will release negative chemicals that travel through your body and can change the shape of the receptors on cells lining your heart, thereby increasing susceptibility to cardiovascular illness. Simply put, positive experiences induce brain cells to expand; negative experiences cause brain cells to shrivel and die.[5] This is intelligent design!

Confrontation Equals Conquest

Eventually I decided to deal with my issues and picked up my prescription—the Holy Bible. Just another book? Hardly! Generations of intellectuals have tried to discredit the Bible. Yet, yearly it outsells every best-seller. The Bible's power rests upon the fact it is errorless, reliable, and the perfect Word of God.

General Robert E. Lee said, "In all my perplexities and distresses, the Bible has never failed to give me light and strength."[6] (See Appendix: The Bible: The Power of God's Word and Thoughts.)

Numerous times I have stumbled across a wounded bird. I usually take it home. If it lets me, I feed the bird by hand until it gets stronger. Then I set it free. Sometimes the bird dies because it won't eat. It doesn't know the food is its life line and source of freedom. The Bible is that nourishment and life-line to us.

Proverbs 4:20–22 speaks about the *living* word of God: "Listen closely to my words. Do not let them out of your sight, keep them within your heart; for they are life to those who find them and health to a man's whole body." According to our Creator, taking care of our heart and controlling our mind (our thoughts) brings freedom and joy and health to our body.

Face the truth. Opening the book of truth may initially hurt or leave you squirming, but *truth frees the soul.* Truth acts as a filter system in our minds, enabling us to truly put off old ways of thinking so we can begin the metamorphic process of bearing the image of our Creator and living out the personality and life God distinctively created for each one of us. Truth has a way of softening our hearts and minds, allowing God to root out the things that choke out life.

But you say, *I don't know if I can do this! I may not like what I find.* Is freedom worth fighting for? It's a lot harder remaining in thought-bondage. Freedom is experiencing the benefits of what God has created you to have. And God has a plan to help you. He gives us the Holy Spirit, the agent of change. It is his job to put this plan into action. We are dependent on him as he guides us into complete truth, through the Scriptures, and away from lies and deception (John 16:13).

The Holy Spirit comes from the Greek word *paraclete* (John 14:16), which means another helper, one who comes along side and consoles, one who intercedes on our behalf, a comforter and advocate. Jesus named him the "Spirit of truth" (John 14:17). He is like our spiritual GPS system.

When Jesus lived as a human, he was completely dependent on the Holy Spirit. The Spirit gave Jesus the knowledge of the will and ways of the Father. As Christians, we have the same Spirit within us. How amazing is that! We hear God's Word through the Holy Spirit. At the same time we must not assume we have no responsibility simply because we are dependent.

Everything you need to live a victorious, joyful, and abundant life is found in the Holy Spirit residing within you (Gal. 5:22–23). Breaking out of the prison of toxic thoughts is a choice. You cannot conquer what you will not confront. Until we submit our lives to the indwelling and all-powerful Spirit, we will never truly learn to lay aside toxic emotions like anger, malice, pride, abusive patterns, jealousy, lying—the things that destroy relationships and our health (James 4:1–10).

Understanding Growth

Jesus Christ, in the flesh, was the mirror image of the invisible Father (see Hebrews 13). He is the healer who will transform you into the person you were created to be. He is the friend who longs to be in a loving, intimate relationship with you. Everything you need can be found in him.

He taught that people who are growing are motivated to change their thinking. As we grow and change, old, rigid thoughts and beliefs—mindholds, break down and cease to work for us, just as an old wineskin breaks if its filled with new wine.

Jesus said, "No one sews a patch of unshrunk cloth on an old garment, for the patch will pull away from the garment, making the tear worse. Neither do men pour new wine into old wineskins. If they do, the skins will burst, the wine will run out and the wineskins will be ruined. No, they pour new wine into new wineskins, and both are preserved" (Matt. 9:16–17).

One of the miracles of the mind is once we learn something it becomes automatic and unconscious called *automatization*. For example, when you first learn to drive a car, you learn to steer, brake, and judge distance, which requires all your attention. In time, it becomes automatic. You pay little attention because it becomes an unconscious action. Our thinking processes are automatic and unconscious.

We develop automatic thinking patterns in childhood. Some of those patterns are distorted and faulty—*automatic toxic thinking* (ATT), which we bring into adulthood. Many of us put up defense mechanisms if we have been hurt in some way, thereby experiencing dysfunctional relationship after dysfunctional relationship.

Reflect: Only by becoming consciously aware of your personal ATTs can you make room for new thoughts and beliefs. This awareness precedes growth, just as a new wineskin flexes with the new wine.

The Biggest Winner

On the hit television show, *The Biggest Loser,* contestants work hard every week to loose pounds in order to stay on the show. A gigantic scale reveals their weight to millions of Americans. Each person knows weight loss doesn't just happen. They have to fight for it by breaking old mindsets and habits and creating new healthy ones. Desperate to meet their goal, they do whatever it takes.

Jesus said, "For everyone who asks receives; he who seeks finds; and to him who knocks, the door will be opened" (Matt. 7:8). Notice we must do something: ask, seek, and knock.

Paul told Timothy, "For this we labor and strive, that we have put our hope in the living God ..." (1 Tim. 4:10). The words *labor* and *strive* tell us becoming Christlike involves more than let go and let God. The Greek word translated *labor* means to work until one is weary. *Strive* literally means to struggle. But we never struggle alone. It is worth every drop of sweat. Playwright George Bernard Shaw expressed this well: "The harder I work, the more I live."[7]

A saying goes, "God feeds the birds but he doesn't throw the food in their nests" (paraphrase of Luke 12:24). God enables us to work to change our mind, our brain, and our heart, but he doesn't do the work for us. Our part requires continually exposing our minds to the Word of God and persistent prayer that the Holy Spirit will give us the desire and power to exercise discipline in all areas of our lives.

You can do this! Take a step and then another step. Let us go right to God himself, with true hearts, fully trusting him to receive us (Heb. 10:22). Keep going! I promise it's worth it. God's Word to you, "Be strong and work. For I am with you" (Hag. 2:4).

It's your turn to respond: "Jesus, I want to go with you. I want to know you better. We tend to become like what we admire and enjoy. Therefore, the more I focus on your glory God, the more I can be changed into your likeness (holiness). I want to think like the daughter you created me to be. I know it may be like a roller-coaster ride but I'm ready and I know you'll be there to catch me if I fall."

Critical Advice: Everyday, before you begin, pray. We have an enemy who will use whatever means possible to distract you—such as your own mind, other people and noise. First, ask the Holy Spirit to open your mind and heart to his voice, teaching and direction. Second, like Jesus and Paul, boldly tell the adversary, "In the name of Jesus Christ get away from me Satan!" (Matt. 4:10; Acts 16:18).

Part One

Understanding How the Past Influences the Present

I the LORD search the heart and examine the mind.

–God Almighty, Jeremiah 17:10

To get something you never had, you have to do something you never did. The will of God will never take you where the grace of God will not enable you.

–Author Unknown

Love the Lord your God with all your heart and with all your soul and with all your mind and with all your strength.

–Jesus, the Gospel of Mark 12:30

A New Creation?

For decades I lived a secret double life. No, I wasn't a stripper by night or committing crimes or having an affair. I was living in my own kind of closet. By day I was a woman who worked hard at making her outside sparkle, hoping others would think she had it completely together. I had the right job, wore the right clothes, and associated with the right people.

As the sun began to set each evening, I retreated into a dark, depressing dungeon where I fought battles with my demons. I held a secret no one could know about. I had lost control over my life. I was a bulimic, a binge drinker alcoholic, soaring on a roller-coaster ride with depression. There was no joy, only fear and shame.

I had become skilled at walking in a counterfeit light, donning a fresh new Cover Girl mask each day. I couldn't take living in the dark any longer. I was one of the walking dead. Then something happened on my way to hell … I got saved. I made a choice to commit my life to Jesus.

However, life was still all about me. I was a saved person but still in bondage. My ego was still on the throne of my life. I continued dressing for success. My addiction to food had miraculously disappeared, but I still desired my wine and continued to indulge myself with unnecessary and overpriced clothes and shoes, cosmetics, and diet supplements. My vocabulary was still "me," "my" and "mine." And office gossip? Count me in! *I had not been set free from myself.*

My thinking and behaviors pretty much remained the same. I had much of my old nature and desires. Underneath my mask I continued to ooze with jealousy and judgment and pride. The same negative emotions that came out of a consumption-fixated culture and the party girl lifestyle still held my soul hostage. In my heart, I desired to be completely free from this way of life, but my brain did not do what I wished. I was torn: God or self? I wanted both. But that was like mixing oil and water—they don't unify.

Something surely went wrong when God got a hold of me, because the Bible says, "If anyone is in Christ, he is a new creation; the old has gone, the new has come!" (2 Cor. 5:17). My old was alive and well, and I certainly did not feel brand new. Did God take a closer look at me and decide I was a lost cause, leaving me to struggle in my own self-made kingdom? *What's wrong with me? I'm so dysfunctional!*

First, the truth is, believers can be in bondage. Second, we all are dysfunctional in one way or other, which you will discover as you journey through this book. People from highly dysfunctional families often think they are a lost cause because they see the family's brokenness as generational and hopeless. The dysfunctional cycle and masked mindset can be broken. It may take professional help.

A pastor or spiritual person may conclude I was an example of a new Christian who failed to stand against Christianity's greatest enemies: the world, my own self, and the enemy, Satan. I was immature, worldly, controlled by my own desires, and dealing with a lot of junk from my past. Their advice: get in line with what God's desires and dethrone my self-centeredness.

If I had sought a physician, he or she would take a family history and complete a medical examination. Based on the exam, the doctor may prescribe anti-anxiety medication. There is a possibility he or she would then refer me to a psychologist who after a few sessions might diagnose me with obsessive-compulsive disorder (OCD), which is a type of anxiety disorder. But I'm still flubbing around in this pit! I start to speculate about the state of my brain.

Many difficult or unnatural behaviors may be related to functional problems in the brain. If you understand better how your brain works, that knowledge can actually give you hope. If a person is unresponsive to psychological or pastoral intervention, or conventional medical science, the next step would be to consider physically evaluating the brain itself through the clinical use of brain imaging (PET, fMRI, SPECT scanning).

Today, with the advent of brain scanning, scientists no longer have to speculate about the brain's role in our personality and decision-making skills. Brain technology has helped many people understand themselves. They learn to forgive themselves for behaviors they really did not want to do. Mom and Dad no longer condemn themselves as "bad parents" when their child is diagnosed with a mood disorder.

Understanding their brain also helps people move beyond the past and into the future God has planned for them, "plans to prosper you and not to harm you, plans to give you hope and a future" (Jer. 29:11). A scan may show overactive brain activity, which has been associated with OCD, which might explain my behavior. I was trying to settle down the pattern of over activity in my brain.

Our Fearfully and Wonderfully Made Brain

Have you ever taken the time to muse over the magnificent complexity of your brain? Most of us don't really do anything to care for it, yet it manages our entire body—every organ and system. It gives us the capacity for art, language, moral judgments, and rational thought. The brain can store more information than all the libraries in the world, which explains why it takes us "mature" folks longer to retrieve data!

The brain responds to our thoughts and behaviors, which determines who we are, our personality. It is responsible for our memories, movements, and how we sense the world. Our moods and feelings originate in our brain, which affects our will to do right or wrong. The female brain responds more intensely to emotion. Feelings, especially sadness, trigger neurons in an area *eight times larger* in the female brain than in the male brain.[8] That explains a lot, doesn't it?

The mind is what the brain does. It's the software running on the hardware of the brain. Right now, it is feeding your understanding with knowledge by translating ink shapes on these pages, speaking them into your mind, and automatically filling them into your memory bank. Our minds can reach into the past through memory or reach into the future through imagination.

Our brain is amazing and reflective of God's greatness. How our brains function likely determines how well we connect with others and how close or how distant we feel from God.[9] Throughout our lives, many of us have received ongoing toxic messages that we're defective in some way. Research suggests abuse in early childhood alters how the brain reacts to stress.[10] Because it is normal for our thoughts to run on automatic, we often end up in repetitive, pain-generating cycles of which we are not even aware.

If there is a physiological reason, being able to view your own brain scan may be a step in the healing process. *I have a medical problem! I'm not so stupid after all.* Recent research indicates we can train our minds, thus change our brains. In most cases, you can change the physiology of your brain, which means you can fix the way you think. However, there are certain people who are resistant to change due to a deep-rooted psychological or biological or spiritual reason, which might require professional intervention.

A Holistic Approach

This is certainly not a black and white issue. Every person is unique. In my particular case, spiritual relationships and pastoral intervention set me on the road to restoration, enabling me to eventually live as that new creation. This is not to say that counseling and medication would not have been beneficial.

The bottom line is there is no inner conflict that is not psychological because our minds, emotions, and will are always involved. Likewise, there is never a problem which is not spiritual because God is always present. And as long as we are living on earth, the odds of being tempted, accused, or deceived by the devil are never ending. If we can accept that reasoning, we will not limit our options to only medical answers or psychological answers. If we want to truly understand ourselves, we should approach the mystery of our human soul from all angles.

We know there is a mind (brain), heart, body, and spirit connection. Multiple studies suggest patients view spirituality as an important dimension in their recovery. Spirituality is a powerful healing tool and can sometimes do what no psychotherapist or formal treatment can do. Often it's the combination of spirituality, therapy, and a solid medical, nutritional, and exercise plan, which are a winning combination.

Studies have also shown that prayer can lead to better health. Researchers started out with approximately four hundred patients recovering from heart problems. Half of the patients received prayer, the other half didn't. According to Dr. Dale Matthews, Georgetown Medical School, patients who were prayed for had half as many complications and a lower rate of congestive heart failure than those who were not prayed for. [11] Other studies have had similar results.

Spiritual or clergy counseling is usually immediate and often crisis-based. Pastors usually cannot help the person unravel years of issues that led to their behavior. Medical science is wonderful, but it cannot detect a spiritually broken heart or help reshape our hearts and minds into one like Christ.

We cannot overlook spiritual warfare. The devil is real. Just because we do not see him does not mean Satan is not working destructively in our lives.

In his book, *Who's Pushing Your Buttons,* psychologist John Townsend stated:

> I have witnessed the supernatural force of demonic influence and believe it is actual, just as it is taught in the Bible. Since one of Satan's strategies is to tempt people away from God, it makes sense there are times that a button-pusher's lack of responsibility, attitude of blame, or denial could have a demonic origin. At the

same time, the Bible teaches a balance of factors. Not every problem has a demon under a rock. But some do.[12]

Dr. Neil Anderson, author of the best selling book, *The Bondage Breaker,* wrote:

> Much of what is being passed off today as mental illness is nothing more than a battle for our minds. To pass this off as some kind of chemical imbalance is to remove the church from the ministry of setting captives free. If all those negative thoughts are just flesh patterns, then why did the thoughts leave when these believers (of the Bible) submitted to God and resisted the devil? Flesh patterns don't instantly leave upon command.[13]

I contend that sound medical and psychological advice cannot be replaced with spiritual care, and vice-versa. Wholeness of health is a journey. All areas need to be explored which is the objective of this book.

Not by Might

Do you truly want to change your thinking and your life? Are you ready to begin to the process of breaking your mask? *Yes!* Jesus taught that wholeness could only be achieved through moving toward God. Start packing your bags and get ready to move out of your comfort zone!

God promises us an abundant life. However, we don't sit around waiting for God to tap us with a magic wand. "The Spirit told Philip, 'Go ...'" (Acts 8:29). We pursue the abundant life promised to us, and the Holy Spirit moves us out. God can't equip us with his power if we're racing around. His spirit won't empower us if we're ignorant to what he is saying. He requires our complete attention before he will fill us with the powerful presence of his spirit.

The Israelites had been exiled in Babylon for seventy years. They had witnessed the strength of the most dominant military power in the world. When the Israelites finally returned home to Jerusalem, they found their city in utter ruins. I imagine a sort of post 9/11. Then came God's Word, "Not by might nor by power, but by my Spirit" (Zec. 4:6). He was telling them the rebuilding would not be accomplished by their own power and resources but by his spirit. As long as they had God's spirit, they had everything they needed to make change happen.

If this journey to tossing out toxic thoughts seems daunting, it will be if you look to your own skills, knowledge, and resources. You will become discouraged. The success of your journey will depend on how well you follow the spirit of God. Remember, no one, not even Satan, can hinder God from carrying out his plan for your life. God's Word affirms, "for you are highly esteemed" (Dan. 9:23). Could there be any words more heartfelt from God than these?

As a believer in Jesus Christ, you have been adopted into his family and hold a brand new position *in him*. It is like marrying into royalty. Your position has changed, which means it is time to change the way you think about yourself … and others. Robert Browning said, "My business is not to remake myself, but make the absolute best of what God made."[14] That is exciting!

Reflect: Name three to five things (objectives) you hope to get out of this book.

The Royal Wedding

When you were a little girl, were you mesmerized with the stories of *Cinderella, Sleeping Beauty,* and *Snow White* as I was? I frequently imagined what it would be like to be rescued by a handsome prince and live happily ever after in elegant gowns. Then I grew up and witnessed the fall of Prince Charming. I realized my palace was really a stable and my job was to clean up after his horse, much like Cinderella's old existence.

How could I be so dumb for believing in a fairy-tale existence? Maybe I wasn't so dumb. Maybe males are wired to fail so there'd be a place in our heart for our Prince—Jesus. Think about it, if all these guys were the real Prince Charming, why would we need Jesus?

Fairy tales may not come true, but when you took Jesus's hand and committed to follow him, your status changed to royalty. You are now his daughter, the daughter of the King, a joint heir with Jesus Christ, chosen of God. To be a "chosen one" is to be uniquely loved as one of Christ's own (Col. 3:12; 1 Pet. 2:9). Soak in this truth. If you don't know who you really are, you won't think or act like God's daughter.

When God chose you, he pulled you out of the mainstream of humanity. He chose to bring you to him so you might be different. God is consumed with the very thought of you! God will not force you to become his, but when you respond, you are called holy one, separate one, and a saint (1 Cor. 1:2). You are unique and beloved by God, which means you are very different from the world. If you don't act different, then you have gone against the very thing God has given you.

Our position has changed. We have been rescued by our prince, and there ought to be an outward manifestation of that change in status. When the clock struck midnight, I doubt Cinderella wanted to go back and live with her wicked stepsisters. Cinderella married the prince, moved into the palace, and lived in elegance with dozens of pairs of glass slippers. Her new life demanded she think and live as a princess.

We don't know how Cinderella's life went, but I imagine either one of two ways. She threw off her old mindset, cutting all ties to her old lifestyle and her Jezebel wicked stepmother and stepsisters. When she looked in her mirror, she saw herself as a princess with a brand new life ahead of her and chose not to look behind.

Or, she had a continual internal war on her hands. Having always been told by her wicked stepmother she was a loser would have been the frontline of her personal, emotional war. Those deadly thoughts would crop up over and over again. *You*

Kimberly Davidson

have no right to be the princess! Once the prince sees you for who you really are, he'll surely dump you. This fairytale life is only temporary because everyone will soon see your ugliness. Left unchecked, Cinderella's thoughts might become an enormous mental mind-hold. All she hears is, "You do not belong."

Eleanor Roosevelt said, "No one can make you feel inferior without your consent."[15] Right now you may feel you have little power here on earth, but you are dead wrong. If you are a believer in Jesus Christ, you belong and you share in his inheritance and his power. Cinderella was the one who fit into the glass slipper. She belonged. We love these fairy tale stories because, in their child-like way, they give all of us hope. Hope that our prince will rescue us. He has. Your position has changed! You belong!

Reflect: Cinderella's new life demanded she think and live as a princess. In an honest conversation with God ask, "Lord, What is it about myself I don't accept?"

The Cost of Losing Our Mask

This change in position does not lead us into a perfect existence. The truth is my new self still lives in my old body (Rom. 7:21–25). Our old nature and ways don't instantly disappear when we become a believer. We don't automatically think all good thoughts and express the right attitudes.

What many of us fail to realize is we don't get an immediate personality overhaul. We are new in Christ but still live in the same world, with the same family, in the same body, with all those old memories, desires, habits, and consequences called the "old self." Becoming a Christians doesn't remove the internal impulse to sin nor does it deter the devil from trying to exploit it. What we have now at our disposal is the enabling power that God offers so we may resist these influences.

As Christians, we are brand new people on the inside. We are not reformed, rehabilitated, or reeducated—we are recreated (new creations), living in vital union with Christ (Col. 2:6, 7).

When we are "born-again" we are beginning a new life under a new Master. We use the words *conversion* and *regeneration* which emphasize our need to anticipate and expect change. This is the great paradox. We are to work diligently on our faith, yet as we walk with God, we are always aware only he can bring about lasting change in our lives.

When our lives begin to change under our new Master, we can expect conflict to arise in three areas of our lives: *spiritual* (warfare with Satan and his demons), within *ourselves* (the old self or flesh), and from *the world* (a system of different or unhealthy set of values and morals). Our minds and hearts are the battleground where conflict with these enemies are either won or lost.

It can be very hard to discern when our struggles are a result of the devil's intervention; us acting in our flesh; environmental stress; cultural pressure; or even abnormal brain physiology. Whatever the origin of the struggle, we know God is actively present. However, the enemy will whisper, *Change is messy, and you'll upset the delicate balance of your family. Leave it alone!* So, your only hope is to live in denial and bury your feelings alive … but they never die!

Don't deny yourself your birthright as a child of God and be satisfied with a joyless life. Confront and conquer the lies! By making certain changes in your thinking and behavior, you can become a new and different person. Faith is often spelled: R-i-s-k.

The starting point is here. "Apply your heart to instruction and your ears to words of knowledge" (Prov. 23:12). "Do not merely listen to the word, and so deceive yourselves. Do what it says" (James 1:22). The Bible, God's holy Word, has the power to transform the human personality. Many people are repelled by the Bible because they believe it is a life of "don't do's." It's actually quite the opposite. It is a life of "to do's." *It is also a* description of who we are in Christ. *Who* you are will shape what you think and do.

The Bible says, "Do not conform any longer to the pattern of this world, but be transformed by the renewing of your mind"

(Rom. 12:2). We must take a closer look at what is filtering through our hearts and minds and ask the tough questions: Why do I act this way? What or who is it that sets me off? When do I seem to be most vulnerable? We want God to reveal the why. Quite often we don't like what we see.

Without a change of mind, our lives will remain as they've always been, no matter what we do or what we try. No matter how many retreats we attend, how many books of the Bible we read, or how often we go to church. If we don't have a mind change, we will still have the same problems and defeats.

When I was in second grade, our family moved from America to England. Nothing was normal any more—new words and accents, a new way of dressing, new sights and sounds, new traditions and values. On the first day of school I had gym class. Unbeknownst to our family, the boys and girls had gym together. Each child was clad in uniform underwear—dark navy blue knickers, or underpants, and a thick, stark white undershirt. I slithered into the gym wearing a flimsy undershirt with a cute little bow and worn out, flowery underpants with a big old hole along the elastic line! The kids snickered and laughed at me. I was devastated. I yearned to go back to America—to the familiar and habitual.

We didn't go back. Mom got me the proper uniform. Eventually I took hold of their customs, finally fitting in. When we are born into the kingdom of God, everything is different. We are different from the world. We learn a new way to think, act, and feel. All the while we are fighting our inner tendencies to do things the old way—to go back. That way is comfortable and takes less effort because it's ingrained in our flesh and programmed into our minds. Sadly, when you become a Christian and move away, the world has a way of laughing and snickering at you.

Reflect: Are you ready to move to a foreign country? What does your answer say about the state of your mind?

Mary Magdalene Set Free

We cannot bring about lasting change in our lives apart from the work of the Holy Spirit. Our relationship should be an intimate partnership. Intimate means we get inside to know another person deeply. This partnership comes out of our actual union with Christ through the work of the Holy Spirit. We *part*ner with him to do our *part*. We are truly participating with Jesus. "I am in my Father, and you are in me, and I am in you" (John 14:20). This is an intimate partnership.

How do we relate to God, a person we never visually see or physically touch or audibly hear? By faith. I know he listens when I speak even though I don't have immediate evidence. The key to experiencing God is to come to him empty, which is hard to do. Coming to God empty feels like we're losing control, and it scares us. But knowing God intimately is the key to everything.

A relationship with God requires the same components that build any relationship. Reveal the real you, show genuine interest in that other person, honor the relationship, and own up to your part of tarnishing or hurting that relationship.

God wants to partner with us to make a difference in this world. There was one woman who partnered with Jesus and made such a difference. This woman took off her mask and embraced a new life. Her name was Mary Magdalene, a woman, like many of us, in search of hope and purpose.

Before meeting Jesus, Mary was a tormented woman. She has been labeled a prostitute, but there is nothing that specifically points to that. When Jesus found Mary, he saw a woman in brutal demonic bondage and in need of a savior.

The symptoms of demonization, or demon possession, in the New Testament were varied. Most often it is was portrayed as an affliction. It was also thought that some demons, while not causing illness, were the cause of what we now call mental disorders. Demons could enslave a person without acutely making them ill. The common element of demonization is that the person involved is being destroyed either physically, emotionally, or spiritually. Thus Jesus directly confronted and cast out unclean spirits. Scripture invariably presents demonized victims with utterly ruined lives.

Demons today represent darkness in our lives. They disguise themselves as stress, anxiety, guilt, rejection, addiction, compulsion, unforgiveness, or depression, things that distract us from the pain. Think carefully about what form demons take in your life today.

No one could help Mary until Jesus came along. He did more than free her from the torment of evil. He changed her from the inside out and set her apart. He took her as a partner in ministry. Scripture also tells us Mary was not the only woman Jesus delivered from torment (Luke 8:1–2).

Restored to her right mind, the bondage broken, she was now a woman filled with love. Her joy came from devoting her life to Jesus' ministry. Our greatest joy is joy in God. Then, on that dark day, Mary was there to witness the crucifixion (Matt. 27:55–56).

It was Mary to whom Jesus first appeared (John 20:14–16; 18), not to the apostles, rulers and kings, nor even his mother. She was the messenger to the apostles, relating the miracle of the risen Christ. She was a woman without hope until God revealed himself to her. Nothing you have done could negate the same kind of touch.

A transformed life is an effective witness to the power of God. However, too many Christians are not experiencing the enjoyment of God's peace and power. Instead of traveling first-class, they travel third class with the cargo, complaining all the way, sadly wasting life. You have the power to choose to change your life and thinking today!

Reflect: Look up and mediate on Colossians 9–14. Imagine that Paul is speaking to you directly.

R.E.S.I.S.T. Recap

Recognize spirituality is a powerful healing tool, but often it's the combination of spirituality, counseling, and a medical plan that are a winning combination to heal toxic thoughts and change your life.

Embrace this new exciting journey of mind renewal through the power of God's truth. You have the ability to train your mind and actually change your brain.

Submit—Commit to learning *how* to submit your struggles, perhaps minute by minute, because they are impossible to conquer in your own strength. Be committed to seeking God's Word daily.

Identify & Interrogate the world you are living in today. Are you traveling first-class, economy, or with the cargo? Are you truly experiencing God and the life he has designed specifically for you?

Set your mind and heart on God. Partner with the triune God: the Father, the Son and Holy Spirit. When God tells you to do something, respond and see what happens! When you are obedient, you will be blessed. It's all about him, not you.

Thank and Praise God! Make praise the innermost part of prayer. Praise God for who he is all he has done for you in every area of your life—physical, spiritual, financial, emotional—all areas of your life.

The Conflict Zones

There's a bumper sticker that says, "Life never seems to turn out the way you think it will 90% of the time." As Christians we hear talk of joy and freedom, but where is it? Why is life so hard? We've got impressive, timesaving computers and gadgets, yet we are over-stressed because there aren't enough hours in the day to do everything we want. Houses are getting larger, but the size of the family is smaller, not only smaller, but increasingly fractured and broken. This is a picture of a people in bondage.

Bondage is the opposite of freedom. Freedom, according to Americans, means I do what it takes to make me happy. I am independent, self-reliant and self-indulgent. A couple won two tickets to Hawaii. The woman was ecstatic, "I get to go to Hawaii twice!" This is not true freedom.

One who is in bondage suffers captivity of some sort. Not literal chains or bars, but in beliefs and behavior. We cannot spend day after day in this world without it affecting our minds, our hearts, and our souls. They become unguarded. Our hearts start to shift away from God. And the ironic thing is the harder we work to become free, the more freedom we seem to lose.

Most often we aren't even aware this is happening. We go about our business believing all is well, but deep down inside something feels wrong. David cried to God, "How long must I wrestle with *my thoughts* and every day have sorrow in my *heart?* How long will *my enemy* triumph over me?" (Ps. 13:2, *my emphasis*). His soul is conflicted.

A major portion of understanding how our past influences the present is becoming aware of the three major influences in our lives and then learning how to resist them. Toxic thinking is influenced by three different, but related, ways: through the *world,* directly through *Satan* and his demons, and through our own *flesh*. These negative influences commonly work together to lead people away from God, negatively affecting our beliefs, thinking, and behavior. These are our *conflict zones*.

Conflict with the World

"The world" touches everyone in many different ways. *Worldliness* is the attitude that places, self, or things at the center of one's aspirations and activities. The Bible equates it with the very embodiment of evil. This concept is found particularly in the writings of John and Paul, and elsewhere in the New Testament.

Secular usually means "belonging to this age or this world." Worldliness, or secularism, is a worldview or lifestyle oriented toward the irreligious rather than the sacred, towards the natural rather than supernatural. It is the ungodly aspects of our culture, peer pressure, values, traditions, what is in, what is uncool, customs, philosophies and attitudes.

Secularism is guilty of having "exchanged the truth of God for a lie, and worshiped and served the creature rather than the Creator" (Rom. 1:25). The world, as presented in John 1:1–18, is all that is opposed to the Word, Jesus Christ. John wrote, "the whole world is under the control of the evil one" (1 John 5:19). These influences contribute to the breakdown of the family, chemical addiction, pornography, and often trigger abuse.

We often use the word *world* interchangeably with the word *culture*. Culture is sometimes used to define the fine arts, but it is best understood as the total pattern of a people's behavior that is learned and grows out of certain ideas or assumptions that we also call a *worldly* or *worldview*. It is in this sense that this word is used in this book.

Jesus describes Satan as the "prince of the world" (John 12:31). One of Satan's strategies is to conform believers to worldliness disabling their call to be ambassadors for Jesus. He is winning. Too many Christians are not all that different from the world. It's been said that many people are willing to be God-centered as long as God is man-centered.

Although believers are told not to be conformed to this world (Rom. 12:2) we nonetheless are influenced by it. Most Christians live in two different worlds: the one on Sunday morning and the one that includes rest of the week. In practice, both worlds clash. Our disposition, temperament and habits are manipulated through the workplace, media and entertainment industries, advertising, the education system, peer groups; world views and philosophies. No doubt our minds are more at risk now than ever.

If we follow the world's ways, we miss God's blessings. Jesus's disciple John said, "Don't love the world's ways. Don't love the world's goods. Love of the world squeezes out love for the Father" (1 John 2:15, Msg). The Apostle James speaks out against befriending the world because to "be a friend of the world is to become an enemy of God" (James 4:4).

Most of us know the story of Noah and the ark (Gen. 5–9). Noah lived in perhaps the most wicked age in history. No one worshipped God. Instead, they worshipped idols and pursued their own sinful pleasures. These people were so wicked that God planned the most complete and drastic act of judgment recorded in Scripture.

Every temptation imaginable was abundantly available to Noah. Nevertheless, Noah did not follow the crowd. I'm sure there were times when he wondered if it was really worth the work of living righteously when no one else did. The day came when his sons had to choose whether they would follow their father. They had to choose whether to believe those around them or trust what Dad said. They chose to join their father.

We can empathize with Noah as we look around our country. We are surrounded by temptation and evil. What will we choose? We often forget our lives have a profound influence on other people—our spouses, family, coworkers, and friends. It is hard to live a righteous life, but we can find assurance in the life of Noah. God will help us fight evil and temptation because he wants to bless us.

Reflect: We should test ourselves and ask, "Am I being shaped more by the secular spirit of the world, or by the Spirit of God?" I challenge you to find time each day to turn the world off. Be still. Come into God's presence. We'll give quality time to a friend, a therapist, a class, a pastor, or a doctor. We'll find time to eat, but we're not very good at giving quality time to God, the one who really nourishes us. It is imperative you find time in your schedule for God.

Idolatry

At the time of Noah, God concluded that every thought and imagination of men's hearts was evil. Today idolatry often centers around our own mental images—images of success, power, youthfulness and accomplishment. Our imagination has always been a fertile field for temptation.

We were created by God for the enjoyment of God. However, instead of God, we often seek significance in ourselves or other socially acceptable things such as our work or appearance, possessions or certain people. For many women, clothing represents who they are. Sadly, the Internet devours people's time, and like stimulants, it numbs the brain's pleasure center![16] How we invest our financial resources tells a lot about what we consider important.

When we begin to worship these things over God, or they become an addiction or an obsession, it becomes idolatry, which God considers a sin (Deut. 4:15–19). Our culture promotes "me first" and then others *if* anything is left over. That's *I-dolatry!* God says one thing, and we say, "I think I will consult a different source of wisdom—me!"

In biblical times, Rome operated the same way. "Hail Caesar! You are king—our god!" Those days are long gone, but our world today is its own Rome. "Hail Dow Jones, hail weekend sports, hail workplace success, hail Republican party, hail beauty makeovers, South Beach diet, Dr. Plastic Surgeon, worthy are you all of my time, energy and effort!"

Idolatry elevates pleasures in things or people above pleasure in God. That is why Jesus said, "Protect yourself against the least bit of greed. Life is not defined by what you have, even when you have a lot" (Luke 12:15, Msg.)

Wealth and possessions can be snares to our souls. Unaware and singing "I've Got to Be Me!" and "I've got to have it," we go along with and accept the values of our culture without checking them against the Word of God to see whether these practices are biblical and right. Paul predicted, "People will be lovers of themselves, lovers of money, boastful, proud, abusive, disobedient to their parents, ungrateful, unholy, without love, unforgiving, slanderous, without self-control, brutal, not lovers of the good, treacherous, rash, conceited, lovers of pleasure rather than lovers of God" (2 Tim. 3:1–4).

The opposite is reverence or obedience, which honors God. He beams like any father would when his children are courageous and choose the right thing to do. He takes pleasure in us when we put our treasure in him. If we are to know a transformed life, there must be a change of mind away from worldliness and idolatry towards God's principles and precepts.

Reflect and pray: "Lord, your Word says, "Guard yourselves from idols" (1 John 5:21, NASB). Search my heart and help me to understand the intent of my thoughts. You desire truth. You know the idols in my life that compete with you. Show me and help me to turn from them and serve you only. In Jesus' name. Amen."

Conflict with Satan

The second influence is Satan himself. There are many popular ideas about this evil spirit being. Some think Satan is not real but rather a personification of the wickedness that abides in the world. Others contend that a human being can be under the control or the influence of spiritual forces such as demons. Many Christians who believe in Satan in general do not identify him as being the enemy of their personal lives. Or, they believe because they are Christian, they cannot be affected. This is a lie.

Paul told the Corinthians he was not unaware of Satan's schemes (2 Cor. 2:11). In C. S. Lewis' classic book *The Screwtape Letters*, the demon Screwtape teaches his young protégé, Wormwood, the art of snaring a new Christian. He writes,

> Our policy, for this moment, is to conceal ourselves ... I do not think you will have much difficulty in keeping the patient in the dark. The fact that "devils" are predominantly *comic* figures in the modern imagination will help you. If any faint suspicion of your existence begins to arise in his mind, suggest to him a picture of something in red tights, and persuade him that since he cannot believe in that he therefore cannot believe in you.[17]

Satan is alive today and has a reinforced army. Scripture is clear the enemy isn't one demon but an entire legion of evil spirits following Satan's commands (Mark 5:1–20). The world is under Satan's control. Although created to serve God, today it is Satan's kingdom. He is able to use it to accomplish his purposes and oppose Christ's. Satan's work is widespread and destructive and God permits his evil activity for the time being.

The unsaved are largely under his authority, however, evil forces are at work using invisible powers to enslave and bind Christians (Eph. 6: 11–18). If Satan doesn't attack Christians, why are we instructed to put on the full armor of God so that we will be able to stand safe against all strategies and tricks of Satan (Eph. 6:1, TLB)?

The mind is Satan's most frequent target of attacks. Scripture supports this. Satan incited David to take a census of Israel (1 Chron. 21:1). Judas's thoughts of betrayal against Jesus came from Satan (John 13.2). When Judas realized what he did, he took his own life. Suicide is a tragically permanent choice to a temporary problem, which I think best describes Satan's modem operandi.

Satan deliberately attacks our thought process which ultimately affects our emotions and physical body. Did you know your body reacts to every negative thought because your brain releases chemicals that make your body feel bad? Surely you've noticed how your muscles tense, your heart beats faster, and your hands sweat when under negative pressure.

Why would Satan attack our minds? Because our minds are the part of the image of God where God communicates with us and reveals his will (Eph. 4:23–24). God transforms ours lives by renewing our minds, which he does through his truth—the Word of God (John 17:17).

Unknowingly, we embrace the devil's mind games and accept them as truth. Jesus said, "The devil was a murderer from the beginning, not holding to the truth, for there is no truth in him for he is a liar and the father of all lies" (John 8:44). Lies are very powerful. If Satan can get you to believe a lie, then he can begin to work in your life to lead you away from God and into sin. His primary motive is the murder of our spirit and body.

When we believe the devil's lie instead of God's words of truth, we are powerless to do what is right. This is why he attacks our minds. Our only defense is the inspired Word of God. Faith in God's truth equals victory; faith in Satan's lies equals defeat and destruction. "The LORD is near to all who call on him, to all who call on him in truth" (Ps. 145:18).

Reflect: Satan's mission is to "TAD" us. TAD refers to these malicious fiery darts Satan shoots at us, darts in the form of temptation, accusation, and deception. Our spiritual lives are under attack everyday. It is a war for our hearts and minds and bodies—our very souls. Our plan must be to make the enemy sorry he ever picked on us! Are you ready to fight for your heart, mind, and soul?

The Fence

As we embark on this journey, many of us will face pressure to return to our old beliefs and life styles. Family, friends, our own ego, and Satan's army will try to pull us back toward living as we did before we met Jesus Christ. That's when we must R.E.S.I.S.T. and choose the right way.

The world's offerings may appear the better choice, but Jesus is the *best* choice. What he offers us is perfect, real, and lasting. You can't say that about a job, or money, a man, or Botox. Satan rules in every inflated ego, every power play, and every manipulative move. He shows up in every rape, robbery, lie, addiction, racial slur, harassment, or church split. Rest assured God will not allow anyone or anything to prevent his children from accomplishing his purposes (his deliberate, preset, divine plan). But, there will be conflict.

We've all heard about people being maimed or killed by a shark attack, so you'd think people would exercise caution in waters that are known to harbor sharks. In Australia, a group of sightseers petted the snouts of sharks during a feeding frenzy on a whale carcass. One of the daredevil tourists was even holding a baby while touching the sharks. They are vicious animals that shouldn't be played with or tempted.

Some people are as cavalier in their attitude toward the demonic. The Bible warns us (Christians) not to give Satan a foothold or a grip. It's an area of our minds over which Satan has jurisdiction, which means we have submitted control of that area, knowingly or unknowingly. I contend that just by the virtue of our sin nature he already has a foothold. We certainly give him a larger area to dominate every time we entertain temptation, evil or the supernatural.

Paul warns us to "avoid every kind of evil" (1 Thess. 5:21–22). I believe we should avoid every form of contact with the supernatural or demonic: astrology, new age paraphernalia such as psychics, demonic movies and music, séances, Ouija, charms.[18]

As Christians we know that no human possesses the ability to access knowledge of future events. God is the only omniscient, all-knowing person there is.

If you don't believe the devil is real, that means he can come in under your radar, like that shark. There is a serious struggle going on between Christ and his followers and Satan and his forces. A fictional story goes: there was a large group of people. On one side of the group stood Jesus, on the other side Satan. Separating them was a fence. Both Jesus and Satan began calling to the people in each group one by one, each having made up his or her own mind to go with either Jesus or Satan.

Soon enough, Jesus had gathered a group of people from the crowd, as did Satan. One man joined neither group. He climbed the fence and sat on it. Then Jesus and his people left, and so did Satan and his people. The man sat alone on the fence.

Then Satan came back (he always comes back).

The man said, "Have you lost something?"

Satan replied, "No, there you are. Come with me."

The man said, "I sat on the fence. I chose neither you nor him."

"That's okay," said Satan. "I own the fence."

There's a bumper sticker that states: *Try Jesus. If you don't like Him, the devil will always take you back.*

Reflect: There are only two states of being: submission to God, which represents good. Or the refusal to submit to anyone, except one's own ego, which automatically enslaves one to the forces of wickedness. Any person who sits on the fence and tries to remain neutral in the struggle between good and evil is choosing to be separated from God (Matt. 12:30).

We also need to be alert against the two extremes. We should not take Satan too lightly, for fear we discount the dangers. Nor should we have too strong an interest in him. Even if the enemy is temporarily given the advantage, we say to him, "You mean evil against me, but God means it for good" (Gen. 50:20, NASB).

Conflict with the Flesh

As dangerous as the world and Satan are, neither is our greatest problem. Our greatest sources of conflict dwell within us, what the Apostle Paul called the flesh (or the old self). Puritan theologian John Owen called it "the enemy of the soul."

Literally, flesh is our physical nature, the muscular and fatty tissue parts of the body, which are separate from our spirit or soul. Figuratively, flesh is equated to our fallen, sinful, and dysfunctional nature (Gal. 5:17; Jude 23)—humanity's natural orientation away from God. The moment we are born, the struggle with our flesh begins because we are born slaves to sin (John 8:34). We are less able to choose right. Until you understand your fleshly nature, conquering toxic thoughts will be hindered. When our flesh dominates the mind, our thinking is compromised (Rom. 8:5).

The flesh is our desires. Desires are good in themselves, such as desires for food, sleep, and sex; desires to achieve and succeed. This is where our opponent, Satan, strikes. He takes advantage of our nature to do precisely what God would not want us to do (James 1:14–15). Keep in mind, most sins come right out of our flesh—they really don't need the help of Satan.

The notion of sin has basically disappeared from American society. The accusation that you have sinned is often said in a joking tone. We use the term when we talk of consuming a huge piece of double fudge cheese cake. Instead of sin, we speak of crime and its symptoms.

Usually our sinful actions stem from an inner urge to fulfill our own fleshly, self-centered desires, which Paul calls "the deeds of the flesh." Do any of these words in Galatians 5:19–21 (TLB) describe what's in your heart?

> When you follow your own wrong inclinations, your lives will produce these evil results: impure thoughts, eagerness for lustful pleasure, idolatry, spiritism (encouraging

the activity of demons), hatred and fighting, jealousy and anger, constant effort to get the best for yourself, complaints and criticisms, the feeling that everyone else is wrong except those in your own little group—and there will be wrong doctrine, envy, murder, drunkenness, wild parties, and all that sort of thing

Today we are less likely than our grandparents to learn about the doctrine of sin. Why is it such an uneasy topic? Like death, it's just unlikable. It goes against what our culture teaches. We don't want to think of ourselves as bad or evil people, even though the Bible teaches that this is what we are by nature. Sin is like a foreign language; many of us just can't grasp the concept of it.

Sin is serious business, and insults God. It always has moral consequences. The solution for overcoming sin is reconciliation with God. When we become Christians, God declares war on the sin—the deeds of our flesh. He came up with an amazing way out. His Son, Jesus Christ, out of his incomparable love, chose to give up his divine godly attributes, and heaven, to become mortal. Jesus took on *literal* flesh, called "incarnation," in order to become a human sacrifice to free us from the bondage of our own *figurative* flesh—our sin. It also enabled him to identify with our difficulties.

Jesus destroyed sin's control over us by giving himself as a sacrifice for our sins. He gives the sinner a writ of pardon. Jesus accepts the sinner unto himself, adopting that person into his family and embraces them as a loving shepherd who has found his one precious lost sheep.

Secondly, the fact that Jesus took upon himself our full human nature is a reminder that to be human is not evil—it is good! One can be released from bondage to sin. It requires a renewing of the mind—the ability of the Word of God to give us discernment, direction, hope, clarity, wisdom, and changed thinking.

Reflect: What aspects of your own behavior are you struggling with at this moment?

Our Metamorphosis

In this world "everything sin touches begins to die, but we do not focus on that. We see only the vitality of the parasite [sin], glowing with stolen life."[19] God's intention is to liberate us from our flesh, sin and the world.

When the Bible talks about a healthy renewed mind and body, originally it was speaking to people who lived in an environment free of chemicals and poisons. The minds of the people in Jesus's day were not over-stimulated by the Internet, television, print media, and subliminal advertising. Their minds were not inundated with the volume of garbage we see and hear today, which begins at a very young age.

For Paul, winning the war for freedom and joy is considered to be transformation through "renewing of the mind" (Rom. 12:2; Eph. 4:23). The word *transformed* in Greek is *metamorphosis,* meaning a change in form. But it means more than just a natural change like that of a caterpillar to butterfly. We must make a break with the past so radical that our minds are filled with the thoughts of Christ himself.

Our minds have to be changed in such a way that the old values, beliefs, and practices are replaced by those which conform to the mind of Christ. Scripture presents us as needing to have our hearts replaced and our minds transformed—our spirits given life (Ezek. 11:19). We don't just say, "Lord, change my mind supernaturally now!" Through the Holy Spirit, God leads our thoughts in the right direction. How?

Great change, according to God's Word, generally comes through studying the Bible: " ...my word that goes out from my mouth: It will not return to me empty, but will accomplish what I desire and achieve the purpose for which I sent it" (Isa. 55:11).

No one is changed by an unread Bible. The Word of God must go through our head and heart if it's going to change our heart and life. Jesus said, "The Spirit gives life; the flesh counts for nothing. The words I have spoken to you are spirit and they

Kimberly Davidson

are life." (John 6:63–64). Freedom according to God means we are dependant on him, his Word.

Reflect: Read Isaiah 55:8–13. What will God's Word accomplish in your life?

Our Condition without Christ

Have you noticed that as a culture we seem to be more fascinated by evil than good? Programming gets progressively more graphic and brutal. Villains are more popular than the heroes. The fastest way to kill daytime soaps would be to rewrite the scripts so the plots dwell on moralities—on marital fidelity!

Our culture has a *National Inquirer* mentality. Ian Fleming claimed that without the seven deadly sins our lives would go flat. Even in the church we enjoy (although we won't admit it) the drama that results from scandal. Playwright Dorothy Sayers suggested anytime you introduce the devil into a cast of characters, you have an instant problem: how to keep the devil from stealing the show.[20]

These are examples of mankind's condition without Christ. The Bible says like sheep, we have *all* gone astray (Isa. 53:6). We think and do sinful things our passions or wicked thoughts lead us into (Eph. 2:1–3).

Christians traditionally set aside the word *sin* for real culpable evil. *Sin* may be defined as disobedience to the known will of God. It is loving the wrong things and may be a matter of act, of thought, of inner disposition. Biblically, sin is not only an act of wrongdoing but a state of alienation from God. It is the breaking of covenant with one's savior.

Sin's capability to pervert is so great that humans can be convinced they are doing God's will when in reality their actions oppose it. In the name of God, two men committed atrocities that rank among some of the worst the world has known. In 1925, Adolf Hitler wrote, "By defending myself against the Jew, I am fighting for the work of the Lord" (Mein Kampf). Osama bin Laden said, "Hostility toward America is a religious duty, and we hope to be rewarded for it by God."

Betty announced her granddaughter's birth, "Rejoice! Another sinner is born!" David understood he was sinful from the time his mother conceived him (Ps. 51:5–6). It took me a long time to get this. I thought, *I never did anything to deserve being born a sinner. This doesn't really apply to me.*

Michelle was born addicted to heroine because her mother shot up during her pregnancy. She was born with a generational and genetic predisposition toward drug addiction through no fault of her own. In grade school Michelle became more and more rebellious and bullying kids. That was her nature. Then she tried a little crack and became addicted. She began to shoplift to support her habit. On numerous occasions she broke into her parent's home, stealing cash and valuables. Naturally, her relationship with her family became strained, and eventually it was severed. Until she cleaned up and changed, she couldn't come home. Then the relationship could be restored.

This is what I have been speaking of. Through no fault of our own, we are born into sin. The Bible says we are born with a depraved mind (Rom. 1:24). Depraved means affected by sin, in everything we do.

Today, what the Bible identifies as sin, we label as addictions or character flaws, or ego or dysfunction, or victimization. Many of us, like our society at large, live in denial of sin. Eugene Peterson paraphrases Jesus' words (John 3:19–21, *The Message*):

> This is the crisis we're in: God-light streamed into the world, but men and women everywhere ran for the darkness. They went for the darkness because they were not really interested in pleasing God. Everyone who makes a practice of doing evil, addicted to denial and illusion, hates God-light and won't come near it, fearing a painful exposure. But anyone working and living in truth and reality welcomes God-light so the work can be seen for the God-work it is.

When we delete the word *sin,* we are saying we prefer to live life in darkness and on our own terms. It is easier to become complacent with God's commands and comfortable in our sin. The process goes something like this:

Something bad happens. I hurt. My flesh wants to do something to reduce the pain. Satan sees an opening. He shoots a dart, perhaps through a liquor advertisement. He says, "Dull that pain. Have a couple drinks."…"You still hurt? Have another drink!"

I will. I want to eliminate this pain.

Now I feel badly—emotionally, physically, and relationally. But I still hurt.

I'm just a loser. I can't do anything right. No normal person does what I do.

Now I hate myself, not my behavior. *I must stop!* However, breaking this cycle comes with a high price tag. I don't have what it takes to do the work, so I won't.

Admitting our own sinful state is step one towards mind renewal. If we leave our sin unchecked, it may eventually destroy us. Deep wounds and sin are often like rotten foods in our refrigerator. We smell the obnoxious odor, but we don't know where the stink is coming from. Only as we allow God to fill us with him will we find where the odor is coming from and see our immeasurable worth and be truly free.

Reflect: In the parable of the good Samaritan (Luke 10:25–37), Jesus's focus was not on human nature as bad. He wanted to provide a model for how to be good. Jesus constantly associated with people who might be considered "bad." But he saw all people capable of having a loving relationship with God. He invited them into relationship with him because that is what gave them the power to be good.

R.E.S.I.S.T. Recap

Recognize that you are in a daily conflict with your flesh, the world, and Satan. Dr. Neil Anderson said, "God won't make you walk in the Spirit, and the devil can't make you walk in the flesh, although he will certainly try to draw you in that direction."[21] Your mind has to be changed in such a way that your old values, beliefs, and practices are replaced by those which are spirit driven and conform to the Word of God.

Embrace new ways and tactics to guard your heart and mind from Satan. Consciously begin to put off any old beliefs and lifestyles that are hindering you from being who you are created to be in Christ.

Submit daily your heart and mind in complete dependency on God in order to understand the intent of your thoughts.

Identify & Interrogate every TAD, any foothold, an idol, or worldly thinking. Ask and depend on the Holy Spirit's guidance to do this.

Set your mind and heart on God. Find a specific time in your daily schedule for God. Shine the light of God's Word on your shadows so the darkness will leave.

Thank and Praise God that absolutely *nothing* can get between you and God's love and his plan for your life.

Deadly Deception

One species of firefly has perfected the art of deception. Hungry and lazy male fireflies have learned to mimic the distinctive flashlight of the female. When a potential suitor comes a courting, the fake female gobbles him up!

It is sobering to realize just how easily and willingly we too can be deceived—about God, about others, and about ourselves. Like the fake firefly, it is even more sobering to be shown that the goal of deception is to bring us to a place where we can be totally devoured or self-absorbed. The truth about deception is it is Satan's most deadly missile.

When we do not believe or rest in our position as a child of God, we open ourselves up to Satan's world of deception. His lies are so powerful. *You're not as pretty or smart as her... You're fat... You won't amount to much... If you were only (this or that) then... You've ruined our lives with your addiction... I wish you were never born.* Many of us believe lies about God. *God will punish me when I sin... He is condemning and unforgiving... God delights in sacrificing what I like best.*

These type of lies fall into four distinctive categories of deceptive warfare.

Psychological Warfare

Every one of us has been raised in a fallen world. Our development is based on genetic predisposition; education and personal learning; internalization of attitudes; values, morals, and beliefs about God, others, and ourselves; and distorted worldviews.

In his book *Search for Freedom,* Dr. Robert McGee explains:

When we are very young, we develop patterns of responding to two worlds: our inner world and the outer world. For most of us, the inner world of our thoughts, dreams, feelings, fears, and imagination is even more powerful than the outer world of people, places, and things. As we move through each world, we encounter pain and pleasure. Although we gravitate toward that which gives us pleasure, pain is usually a much greater motivator. This is especially true of emotional pain. The way we respond to emotional pain creates important behavioral patterns we have. It is, in fact, these patterns that create the core relationship problems in our lives.[22]

As we're growing up, the people around us teach us life: who we are, who we trust, what's good or bad, right or wrong, how valuable we are, and generally, what life and this world is all about. Tamara learns who she is from how other people treat her. Her father's desertion taught her a lie: "If I was a better kid, Dad wouldn't have left. If I was lovable and important, he would have stayed and Mom wouldn't hurt so bad."

We become deceived when we choose to believe messages that do not line up with the Word of God. Lies wreak havoc on our minds and hearts. Haven't we all fallen to the temptation of envy because we believed someone else had what we needed? Haven't we all failed to resist the pull to retaliate against someone who hurt us? Haven't we all met someone, perhaps a handsome guy or a slick salesperson, we thought was wonderful, only to discover we were deceived? I did and almost married him! We tend to believe those whom we do not know because they have never deceived us.

Spiritual Warfare

Every addiction, every felony, and every adulterous affair started with one deceptive lie. We are deceived when we believe we are not sinners. Before we sin, while Satan is tempting up, he

Kimberly Davidson

whispers, *No big deal! You can get away with this.* After we sin, his laughs. *Idiot! You'll never get away with this.* Sin gives Satan claim to us. The prophet Isaiah said sin bewitches the soul, making the soul call evil good and good evil, bitter sweet and sweet bitter, light darkness and darkness light (Isa. 5:20).

False teachings are another way Satan gets us to move away from God. Spiritual deception is not new. False teachers may present pieces of God's truth but mixed with untruth. They use "good" as a means to a different end. New Age religion is an example. The emphasis is often on self-sufficiency: "You have the power within." Jesus has warned believers for centuries that many counterfeit prophets will appear and deceive countless people (Matt. 7:15; 24:11).

The Bible tells us not all spirits are from God. Some spirits are demonic, deceitful, and try to mislead us (1 Tim. 4:1). More and more Christian women are being seduced deeply into the New Age worldview of Christianity. On a desperate quest to find answers to the angst in their soul, these alleged truths come from a variety of sources that compliment one another. They are so intriguing and appear life changing. However, they come from one source—the deceiver, Satan. The Bible says, "What good will it be for a man if he gains the whole world, yet forfeits his soul?" (Matt. 16:26).

False teachers divide churches. The source of conflict is usually about who's in charge. Getting our way and knocking down this opponent becomes the main driving force. Satan just laughs as we bicker among ourselves because he is getting his way.

False teachers develop cults and plant new churches that are not based on doctrine, but on feelings. The Bible warns, "See to it that no one takes you captive through hollow and deceptive philosophy, which depends on human tradition and the basic principles of this world rather than on Christ" (Col. 2:8).

Our first line of defense against theological error is a thorough knowledge of the truth. King Solomon used the expression "store up my commands" (Prov. 2:1; 7:1). The idea is to lay away God's truth, our ammo, in anticipation of a future need. Scripture enables us to evaluate and discern sound doctrines that are being taught.

Can you support what you believe using the Word of God? When false doctrines are presented, how will you know they are false unless you know what is true? Those who are not disciplined in learning and pursuing God's Word become targets for cults, New Age influence, and other false prophets. They have no means to evaluate whether they are of God or not. Don't be afraid to ask questions. True teachers will always be willing to give straightforward answers.

Biological Warfare

Today we know that health is far more than mere physical well-being. Roots of illness are found in all aspects of our lives. Studies reveal a mind, body, and soul connection. The workings of the *physical* affect the function of the *mental* and *emotional* and the *spiritual*.

According to a survey by the American Psychological Association, when women are stressed they cope by opting for unhealthy habits. The most common are eating (39%); shopping (25%); smoking (17%); drinking (15%); and gambling (4%).[23] Compulsive overeating may lead to heart disease, diabetes, and certain cancers. ["Stressed" spelled backwards is "desserts."] Smoking can lead to lung cancer, heart disease, or low birth-weight infants. Drinking alcohol in excess may result in cirrhosis or mouth cancers. Gambling and erratic shopping may result in debt or financial ruin which leads to anxiety and ulcers.

Emotionally, if we are depressed or chronically unhappy, we may experience an increased resistance to infection or cancer. Socially, if we lack close ties with others, the incidence of mental illness, respiratory disease, complications of pregnancy, and early death (from numerous causes) may result.

Spiritually, if we are a fatalist, we probably won't seek any type of care. Or, if we feel guilty all the time because of our sin, we put unneeded stress on ourselves, which affects our body. Deception affects our entire lives negatively.

How do we fight back? Worship, prayer, and meditation decreases blood pressure and mental stress and increases hardiness.

Cultural or Social Warfare

In our culture it is not uncommon to lie; in fact, in certain circles it is expected. One company advertised: *Top Lie Detector Polygraph Examiners. Prove your truthfulness or find out if your suspicions are right.* David attested that "Everyone lies to his neighbor; their flattering lips speak with deception" (Ps. 12:2). A great deal of Scripture speaks to deception because it is so common and part of our world.

We deceive ourselves, especially when we think we are more important than others and certain rules don't apply to us. Jesus would say, "We think we won't reap what we sow." Pride is a spiritual cancer that affects every part of our lives. We may work to overcome our pride—go into pride remission—but it will eventually resurface. Satan constantly dangles the bait of vanity, self-importance, conceit in our face because pride has the potential to destroy our lives and ministry.

I personally think *denial* is our culture's greatest deception because it is deliberate self-deception. Christian psychologist Les Carter agrees: "The Number One trait that hinders individuals from making personal improvements is denial. We each hate feeling like we are being exposed as inadequate, and so in self protection, it seems easier to simply say our problem does not exist."[24]

We unconsciously push aside or repress what needs to be exposed, creating a deeper mindhold. It's a commitment to our heart to never be hurt again, a refusal to face facts, and a way to break the feeling of powerlessness. There are consequences.

Reflect: Jesus said, "Watch out that no one deceives you. Therefore be as shrewd as snakes and as innocent as doves. Be on your guard" (Mark 13:5). How do we begin to break the cycle of denial? Pray first, asking God to help you listen acutely. Be willing to hear another's perspective. Trust that others can see blind spots that you cannot see in yourself. Second, battling deception requires identifying and then taking these deadly thoughts captive to Jesus Christ (2 Cor. 10:5).

My Deal with the Devil and the Culture

Ophelia, in Shakespeare's *Hamlet,* illustrates the destructive forces affecting young women. Ophelia is a typical girl, footloose and fancy-free. But she loses herself in adolescence. She falls in love with Hamlet and lives only for his approval. She doesn't have a relationship with God and the insight of the Holy Spirit to guide and direct her, so she lives merely to meet Hamlet's and her father's demands. Who she is, her value, is determined solely by their approval, and she is torn apart. She goes mad with grief. Elegantly dressed, tragically she drowns in a stream filled with flowers.

For twenty years I lived an Ophelia existence. I attempted to take control of my mind, yet I couldn't conquer the addiction to food, alcohol, cigarettes, diet pills, and my promiscuous behavior. Unconsciously, I believed Satan, who, disguising himself as an angel of light, had what I was searching for—love, beauty, and success. It was only after I submitted my brokenness, and what memories I had, to God that he helped me pinpoint how I ended up in this dungeon, thus starting the breaking down of mindholds.

As a kid, our family moved quite a bit. The first major move was age seven, moving from America to London, England. I was teased by schoolmates because I didn't fit into the culture. I was unlike them because I had an accent. I felt stupid because I needed a tutor. I was weird because my clothes were different. What I heard was, "You do not belong."

You never get used to other kids being mean, but in time you learn how not to feel the sting of rejection so much because of a deep-seeded desire for acceptance. A message such as "She's a weirdo," or "Honey, looks like you haven't skipped a meal," says to the child, "You are not accepted."

We moved back to America when I was twelve. *Again* I was weird and different, but now I was entering adolescence—the hurricane years. Further rejection and teasing from schoolmates only made the previous mindholds deeper. The pain of rejection became part of my normal thought process.

Rejection is one of our most powerful and destructive emotions. It may cause as much distress in the pain center of the brain as an actual physical injury, according to research. Rejection feels like pain to the brain. Perhaps this is why we use the term "hurt feelings." One of the studies' authors said, "While everyone accepts that physical pain is real, people are tempted to think that social pain is just in their heads, but physical and social pain may be more similar than we realized." [25]

I expected people not to like me so I worked tirelessly trying to conform to the way I thought my peer group and teachers wanted me to be. And today it's not much different. Young girls experience a great deal of pressure from the culture to create a false self, a mask. This disorients and depresses many girls because they feel the pressure to be someone they're not.

We moved several more times. Moving can be painful. It's a loss. Moving stresses both parents and children, especially if the move is resented. The loneliness and loss of friendships hurts. Research shows that loneliness can affect the body's immune system. Many are at risk for depression, and relocations increase the risk of teen sexual activity. It's their way of gaining social acceptance. [26]

I fell in with the wild crowd, feeling the pressure to fit in. I smoked cigarettes and tried alcohol and drugs. This group gave me a sense of belonging and a means to forget the rejection and losses. Then I began to gravitate into a new world of worshipping celebrities and models. I believed the lie that to be popular you have to look like a model. Teen magazines say, *Don't worry about being good, worry about looking good and being socially accepted!*

Girls will react to the cultural pressures to abandon their real selves. The result: many withdraw, get angry, or depressed. "Fat talk" flourishes. Something mysterious happens to girls in adolescence. They enter their own Bermuda Triangle, crashing and burning as they navigate through social and physical development. They sell their souls for popularity, becoming their own version of a Cover Girl.

I pretty much turned off my God-given talents and gifts in search of the Western culture's definition of ideal. I decided I was going to be a super model. A few boys in my sixth-grade class laughed. "Yeah, for *MAD Magazine*." Satan then murmured, *You're ugly, girlfriend. Give it up!* I didn't give it up. I'd do anything to be a beautiful super model or celebrity. And why not? In this culture beauty has its rewards. This was the beginning of the Cover Girl masquerade.

Reflect: In what specific ways do you relate to the author's story? Have you rejected your true identity—the person God created you to be? Explain.

Image Management

Psychologist Mary Pipher says, "Girls become 'female impersonators' who fit their whole selves into small, crowded spaces. Girls stop thinking, *Who am I? What do I want,* and start thinking, *What must I do to please others?* American culture has always smacked girls on the head in early adolescence."[27]

My main concern was my own image management. As I grew into early adulthood, my self-esteem continued to deteriorate. (I never realized how universal my experiences were.) I started binge drinking regularly in college. It was great because my insecurities vanished. But clearly, I was self-medicating— the stress, anxieties, and pain. And then my body started desiring and needing the alcohol.

Alcohol abuse usually leads to inappropriate sexual behavior. I couldn't stop the promiscuity. I did what I thought I should do in order to be accepted. Again, I justified it. *Everyone else is sleeping around.* It was a way to fill the hole in my heart. But it only deepened the wounds of shame, humiliation, and abandonment.

Sex is portrayed as something fun without consequences. I was playing Russian roulette, and it was worth the risk. I eventually got pregnant and chose to have an abortion. When you are promiscuous, you eventually feel used and abused. Whether you enter into it willingly or have it forced upon us, sexual sin causes severe wounds which require healing. Using the Cinderella analogy again, Cinderella didn't take her clothes off to win her prince. When the clock struck midnight and she returned home, she didn't lose anything she couldn't get back the next morning!

Scripture says the person who lives for pleasure is dead even while she lives (1 Tim. 5:6). My soul was dead. There was nothing to me. If you were to take off my mask, there would be no face. A person without a face is indifferent. I didn't care about others. I used people. It was all about me.

Friends called me on my behavior. My response, "I was drunk." In other words, *I'm not accountable for my actions. Dysfunction made me do it!* Charles Colson wrote, "Making excuses is part of human nature; because of our excuse making, we now live in a society filled with victims and nonjudgmental authorities. Mystified I wondered, "Why is this happening me? I am basically a good person. Why do I keep falling into this hole [temptation]? I never asked this evil monster into my life. Not fair! What's was wrong with me [accusation]?"

There was no joy, no hope; only fear and self-condemnation. The shame kept feeding every destructive behavior: the bulimia, drunkenness, and promiscuity, which continued to feed the shame, paralyzing my soul in a never-ending battle, a battle which I had no control over. I hated myself and tried to cover up with success, gossip, and materialism. Asking for help meant admitting I was a failure. People would know I was a phony, which is pride. So I became the "The Master of Secrecy" [deception].

Reflect on Dr. Mary Pipher's evaluation. It is gripping:

> Most women struggled alone with the trauma of adolescence and have led decades of adult life with their adolescent experiences unexamined. The lessons learned in adolescence are forgotten and their memories of pain are minimized. They come into therapy because their marriage is in trouble, or they hate their job, or their own daughter is giving them fits. Maybe their daughter's pain awakens their own pain. Some are depressed or chemically addicted or have stress-related illnesses—ulcers, colitis, migraines, or psoriasis. Many have tried to be perfect women and failed. Even though they followed the rules and did as they were told, the world has not rewarded them. They feel angry and betrayed. They feel miserable and taken for granted, used rather than loved ... the years fall away. We are back in junior high with the cliques, the shame, the embarrassment about bodies, the desire to be accepted and the doubts about ability. So many adult women think they are stupid and ugly. Many feel guilty if they take time for themselves. They do not express anger or ask for help.[29]

Inside the Lion's Den

Jesus did not come into the world to condemn it (John 3:17). He didn't want people to feel bad about themselves. He wanted people to feel loved by God. Jesus wanted people to find freedom from shame and self-condemnation, not get stuck in it.

Cleansing your thought process is to rid your mind of self-condemnation, guilt, fear, and shame. Shame is not an easy subject. Most people choose to ignore it because it usually is a result of exposure of sin or some perceived defectiveness. If my lifestyle—my sins—were exposed, I would have been mortified.

Naively, I had made a deal with the devil. By believing his

lies and living a sinful life, I gave him a foothold, a place in my mind and heart to unpack his bags and set up a dungeon. Peter warns us, "Your enemy the devil prowls around like a roaring lion looking for someone to devour" (1 Pet. 5:8). His goal is to destroy our minds, hearts, bodies, and spirits, in one way or other.

Satan's number one motive is to shatter our relationship with God and deny God his due glory, honor, and praise. He'll try to demolish your character even though you did not do anything to bring on his attack. Satan's purpose is to make you ignorant to God's will. He attacks God's Word because it reveals God's purpose and plan for our lives. Apart from the Word, we have no sure way of understanding the will of God. The will of God is his expression of love for us. It establishes our true identity—who we really are.

God's will is not a duty as Satan would have you believe. He plants the lie, *If you choose to follow God's will, you'll have to give up everything you enjoy!* When we're out of God's will, we make bad decisions and live recklessly. Sadly, we influence others.

Paul, too, saw his enemy as a lion, but he knew where to find refuge. "The Lord stood at my side and gave me strength ... and I was delivered from the lion's mouth. The Lord will rescue me from every evil attack and will bring me safely to his heavenly kingdom. To him be glory for ever and ever" (2 Tim. 4:17–18).

One of the greatest lions in our jungle today is the fear of rejection. Greater awareness of your fear of rejection will result in mind change and growth. Does fear of rejection control your life?

1. Do you feel that it is better not to ask rather than hear "no"?

2. Do you have trouble speaking up for fear of ridicule?

3. Do you often avoid controversial conversation topics that require you to participate and make a stand? Do you automatically assume you will be rejected if you say anything disturbing?

4. Do you avoid the opposite sex because you are worried about being turned down or diminished?

5. Do you ever wonder how different your life could be if you were not afraid of rejection, if you could open up and find out whether your assumptions are correct?

It takes courage to face the darkness and fear of rejection and shine light on it. We need to have the courage to say no to others when they trespass on our well-being and stand alone when others erode our beliefs. Sometimes we have to be the one to reject someone who is hurtful and judgmental such as a boss, family member, or spouse. Sometimes we have to reject a friend who is self-absorbed and disregards our boundaries.

Reflect: If you answered yes to any of these questions, ponder these suggestions. With the Holy Spirit's assistance, interrogate where these feelings of rejection are coming from and begin to replace the toxic thoughts with God's promises about you.

- Recognize your need to please and accommodate others. Is there a pattern?

- Rehearse in your mind the confrontation where you feel you risk rejection. See the whole scene through to the end. Pray and imagine a successful outcome.

- List each compliment you receive every day. Note whether you resisted or accepted the compliment. What did the compliment say about who you are?

- Give yourself permission to say no. Balance your available time with your energy level. Say no to the energy vampires. They will respect the new you.

- Each week stretch yourself beyond your comfort zone. Ask for something that places you at risk. It gets easier with practice and prayer.

Saving Ophelia

Like Ophelia, I was in danger of drowning. It was beginning to look like a life or death situation. It was vital I be revived. I needed someone to point me to Jesus Christ. "In my distress I called to the LORD; I cried to my God for help. From his temple he heard my voice; my cry came before him, into his ears" (Ps. 18:6).

God sent that person and he took me to church. Jesus walked into my messed up life and a couple months later I was saved. The Bible says, "That if you confess with your mouth, 'Jesus is Lord,' and believe in your heart that God raised him from the dead, you will be saved" (Rom. 10:9). Jesus died to save his people from their sins (Matt. 1:21).

Jesus pronounced, "Daughter, You're free to go. I've done the time for you (Acts 2; 2 Cor. 3:17). Now go and tell the world what you have experienced." The shackles melted. Evil evaporated.

In the heavenly realm, God shouted, "Hey angels, my daughter has been found! Rejoice, angels!" (Luke 15:7).

Jesus will always meet us right where we are at. We don't have to be good enough, smart enough or religious enough to earn an audience with him. We can have a personal, intimate relationship with *the* God Almighty.

The Bible says when we accept Jesus Christ as our Savior, God sprinkles our hearts with Jesus's blood to cleanse us from a guilty conscience and our bodies have been washed with pure water (Heb. 10:22). He has internally cleansed us from sin. Our consciences that have held onto piles of guilt and shame are clear and cleaned out.

We get an internal extreme makeover. A staple subject of talk shows, makeovers are popular subjects. Today, computer software and online tools are used to create *Virtual Makeovers.* When we think of an "extreme" makeover, we usually associate it with cosmetic or gastric bypass surgery, or the implantation of dental veneers. No external makeover can compare to the internal makeover we receive from Jesus Christ. External makeovers create Cover Girl masks. Jesus washes away the mask.

Our identity changes because he adopts us into his family. Our hearts and minds are cleansed completely, not partially or temporarily (Heb. 9:14). God took all my guilty acts and thoughts, and placed them on Jesus. At that moment, he said, "Kimberly, you are forgiven. Every offense is wiped from your record." God forgives and forgets—completely, and we became righteous—perfect before God.

God took the sinless Christ and poured into him my sins. Then, in exchange, he poured God's goodness into me (2 Cor. 5:21). What a trade! God did more than delete my bad record. He declared me as righteous as his Son! The writer of Hebrews declared, "Their sins and lawless acts I [*God*] will remember no more" (Heb. 10:17). This is the most incredible truth. God now sees me in Christ. I can enter God's presence with boldness!

Jesus now dwells within me and he cannot coexist with that old me. It would be like putting a wild lion in the same kennel with a domestic kitten. The old me wants to fulfill the desires of her selfish heart. She wants the external makeover. But Jesus wants to renew her mind, changing her heart from herself to him and others. That explains why it is so hard for many believers to continue hanging out with their unbelieving friends. They no longer think alike and find it hard to coexist. Darkness cannot coexist with light.

Reflect: Remembering that our old sinful life is dead gives us a powerful motivation to resist toxic thinking and sin. When those negative thoughts or behavior start to creep back in, we can now consciously choose to treat those desires as if they were dead (Col. 2:11–12). What one way might you begin to do that immediately?

Our New Birth

Too many of us live with the idea that something is missing, which often leads to making bad choices, failure, and sadness in our lives. We may become angry or bitter at someone for not being to us what we need them to be. When we ask Jesus to become our Lord, we become complete in him (Col. 2:9). Complete forgiveness. Complete love. Complete peace. Complete victory.

Since the fall, God has been in the business of restoring mankind. Out of God's love, grace is given to sinful people with the promise that, in spite of their inability to keep any of God's commandments, he forgives their sin and accepts them as his children. Grace is not simple leniency when we sin. Grace is power! It is an enabling gift of God not to sin. It is the power to press on—thinking and doing what is right.

Before Jesus, my heart and thoughts were dark, like a cancer which left undetected would have infiltrated and eventually killed me. After letting Jesus in, my spiritual heart turned from darkness to gold, as if the cancer had been removed from my soul. "God has poured out his love into our hearts by the Holy Spirit, whom he has given us" (Rom. 5:5). My commitment to God was (and still is) written on my heart. Jesus set me free from my old evil desires. *I do matter! I'm going to make a difference!*

A lot of the old, bad stuff was wiped out, but not all of it. I no longer had the urge to binge and purge everyday which was a miracle. Many secular mental health professionals call this rare event "natural change" or "spontaneous remission," and some even claim no one can ever recover from an eating disorder.

[Research shows many addicts who fail traditional treatment programs are able to free themselves from their addictions when they develop a connection with God. God can set someone free instantaneously if he so chooses, although we usually see the more traditional path of lots of hard work and therapy!]

God loves to meet and embrace us in that place of broken-ness. Jesus is the only one who can spiritually remove the cancer, changing our heart from darkness to gold with his love. We experience a new birth, a renewal, a transforming resuscitation called *regeneration*. It is an impartation of new life, the theme within the Bible.

"Those who have a sure hope, guaranteed by the Spirit say, "Outward appearances will no longer be our standard in judging other men. Our lives are all controlled by the Spirit now, and are not confined to this physical world that is subject to corruption" (St. Cyril of Alexandria).[30]

Fact: God wants to reweave your life because you have great value. Because he created you, he wants to have a personal relationship with you (John 3:16–17).

Fact: There is something that blocks that relationship with a holy and perfect God—sin. We can't help it, we're human. People are sinful (Rom. 3:23). In this culture, we have exchanged the glory of God for something else: the glory of a bigger house or car or high-powered job or super computer or vacation; whatever makes us tick more than the wonder of God. That kind of glory separates us from our Father. When we begin to interrogate why we want these things, our eyes are opened to the errant motivation behind the why, such as pride or jealousy.

We respond by asking Jesus into our life, believing he is the Son of God. We turn toward God and away from our present way of thinking and living. We begin the exciting adventure of letting God direct our lives and break down those mindholds.

Being a Christian doesn't guarantee we'll never experience pain. When I thought he didn't care about my pain, his Word told me he catches each tear and shares my pain. Today I can say there is no high like *the Most High!*

Jesus came to provide the means by which we can have that fellowship. If we reject Jesus Christ and refuse to be "born again" of God's Spirit, we will not be received into heaven (John 3:5–7).

The messages in this book are directed to those who have embraced Jesus as their Savior. Do you want Jesus to be your Savior? If you are unsure of your relationship with God, deal with that now.

Pray this prayer (simply talk to God):

"Dear God, If I have allowed the world to diminish who you are, let me now see the truth. I know my sin has separated me from you. Thank you that Jesus Christ died in my place and is giving me eternal life. I confess I am a sinner. Jesus, forgive my sin and come into my life at this very moment. Please direct my life. In Jesus's name. Amen."

Congratulations! God has just crucified your old rebellious nature and replaced it with a new loving nature (Rom. 6:6; Col. 3:9–10). Your best life is ahead of you!

Warning: Satan will tell you that because of your past you don't have what it takes to make your life count for the kingdom. Another lie! Send Satan away and counteract that thinking. "I praise you, God, for Jesus and the gift of salvation by faith. To you, Lord God, be the glory!"

Reflect: Close your eyes and picture your life as tapestry. What does it look like? Imagine now the needlepoint being unraveled piece by piece. Picture the most beautiful tapestry on display. It is slowly and meticulously being rewoven by God. He is reweaving this special piece of cloth, your life, to his design.

R.E.S.I.S.T. Recap

Recognize the intense psychological, spiritual, biological, and cultural warfare that is present in your life today, but do not fear it.

Embrace what the Holy Spirit is preparing to show you— old thinking and junk hiding in the crevices of your heart and mind. How ready are you?

Submit your messed up life in prayer. Jesus will meet you right where you are at. Submit any footholds or deals you may have made with the devil as you ask God to reveal them.

Identify & Interrogate—Pray Psalm 139:23–24: "Search me, O God, and know my heart; test my thoughts. Point out anything you find in me that makes you sad, and lead me along the path of everlasting life."

Set your mind and heart on God. He sees you in Christ. Now look at him for exactly who he is, your Father of grace, mercy, and love. Go and tell the world what you are experiencing and learning.

Thank and Praise God that when you were saved, your shackles melted and evil evaporated. "The Lord will rescue me from every evil attack and will bring me safely to his heavenly kingdom. To him be glory!"

Serpentine Seduction

A story goes that Satan called a worldwide convention. In his opening address to his evil angels, he said, "We can't keep Christians from going to church or from reading their Bibles and knowing the truth. We can't even keep them from conservative values. But we can keep them from forming an intimate, abiding experience in Christ.

"If they gain that connection with Jesus, our power over them is broken. So let them go to church but steal their time so they can't gain that experience in Jesus Christ. Angels, distract them from gaining hold of their Savior and maintaining that vital connection throughout their day!"

"How shall we do this?" asked his evil angels.

"Keep them busy in the nonessentials of life and invent schemes to occupy their minds. Tempt them to spend and spend, and then, borrow and borrow. Convince the wives to go to work and the husbands to work six or seven days a week, twelve hours a day, so they can afford their lifestyles. Keep them from spending time with their children. As their family fragments, their homes will offer no escape from the pressures of work.

"Over stimulate their minds so that they cannot hear God's still small voice. Entice them to listen to non-Christian radio whenever they drive, to keep the TV and their DVDs and CDs going constantly. This will jam their minds, breaking that union with Christ. Pound their minds with the news twenty-four hours a day. Invade their lives with every kind of promotional offering, free products, services, and false hopes.

"In their recreation, let them be excessive. Have them return from their recreation exhausted, disquieted, and unprepared for the coming week. Send them to amusement parks, sporting events, and concerts. When they meet for spiritual fellowship, involve them in gossip and malice so they leave with troubled consciences and unsettled emotion.

"If they get involved in soul-winning, crowd their lives with so many causes they have no time to seek power from Christ. Soon they will be working in their own strength, sacrificing their health and family unity for the good of the cause" (Author Unknown).

This is a powerful illustration of what results when our thoughts and actions are left unchecked. It's been said we have created an ADD type society. We are busy, stressed, and distracted. We are in bondage to our cell phones and email.

Reflect: Commit to funnel this energy into following Christ:

1. Read Jesus's Beatitudes (Matt. 5:1–11). He set forth some profound truths, clearly explaining the kind of life that brings us joy and is pleasing to God. Satan's beatitudes bring us down and overload our minds, separating us from our loving Father.

2. Paul said to "put on the full armor of God so that you can take your stand against the devil's schemes" (Read Eph. 6:11–18). Each piece of armor is a characteristic of the Lord Jesus. Anything I do to make myself more like Jesus is putting on the armor of God. Then I am victorious!

Meet Your Enemy

In 1978, some nine hundred members of the People's Temple cult committed mass suicide by drinking a mixture of grape Kool-Aid laced with Valium and Cyanide. These poor souls never imagined that joining this group for spiritual growth and social justice would end in suicide. A University of Oregon commentator responded, "The sad truth is that they had already drunk the Kool-Aid long before they took their own lives, by killing off their ability to think critically and independently. Humans are endowed with extraordinary powers of observation and analysis, and yet we are also susceptible to deep-seeded desires for acceptance and conformity."[31]

This is a picture of Satan at work. What do we really know about this evil creature and his demons? It is interesting to me that there is little in the Old Testament about Satan and his demons. But as soon as Jesus comes on the scene in the New Testament, there are numerous Scripture references about the demonic. When Jesus was born, Satan's power and control were disrupted.

Satan is the name given to the chief of the fallen angels. In Hebrew his name means to be or act as an adversary.[32] The most common Greek word for him is devil, adversary or accuser. As his name indicates, he is engaged in opposing God, his creatures and the work of Christ.Scripture reveals that evil appeared in heaven before it entered the world (3; John 8:44; Rev. 12:9; 20:3). Isaiah 14 paints the picture for us: Lucifer, the archangel, stood at the right hand of God, exercising full authority of the Father in the affairs of creation. No higher position existed. He was an angel of the highest rank, created to glorify God, clothed in beauty and power, and allowed to serve in the presence of God. Lucifer's power and authority were only exceeded by the Creator himself.

Isaiah's story accounts a violent ending of the relationship between Lucifer and the Father (Isa. 14:13–14). Lucifer bellowed, "I will make myself like the Most High!" I bet the heavens thundered and roared that day. Blinded by pride, he actually thought he could seize control from the Almighty God. There were consequences. He was "brought down to the grave, to the depths of the pit" of hell.

Lucifer was rejected. His name, which means Morning Star or Light-Bringer,[33] was changed to Satan and he set up an empire of evil. His mission was to continue roaming the earth disguised as an angel of light (Job 1:7; 2 Cor. 11:14). His goal is to deceive, tempt, and destroy man. Since that dark day, he has hit others with the fiery dart of pride and rejection, hoping they will make the same mistake and rebel against God.

What triggered this reaction in Lucifer? His fall is a mystery. Whatever it was, the result was Lucifer's expulsion from heaven, along with a significant number of angels, who chose to follow him (angels, too, have been given free will). His work is augmented by one-third of the angelic host (Rev. 12:4; 9).

The biblical account of Satan is not unlike the original *Star Wars* trilogy. Darth Vader is the primary antagonist, a dark, ruthless figure out to capture, torture, or kill the films' heroes to prevent them from thwarting the Empire. In our day-to-day lives, two parallel histories occur: one on earth and one in heaven. Everyday we are in positions where we must choose between good and evil.

Satan is a created being with limitations. He is not the opposite of God. He is the opposite of the archangel Michael. Even though Satan is the "god of this world," he is not omnipotent, omniscient, omnipresent, or anything else that characterizes God. C.S. Lewis calls him *God's Satan*—a creature of God who can be really wicked only because he comes from the shop of a master and is made from the best stuff—a superhuman spirit.[34]

Capable of great evil influence, he is ultimately a dog on a leash. Satan has already been defeated through the death and resurrection of Jesus (John 12:31; Col. 2:13–15). "He became flesh and blood by being born in human form; for only as a human being could he die and in dying break the power of the devil who had the power of death" (Heb. 2:14, TLB). When Jesus drew his last breath on earth he said, "It is finished." Satan was also finished. Jesus is the permanent ruler of the whole world. Satan is only the temporary ruler of the part of the world that chooses to follow him.

Evil will still have temporal victories. Satan can never rob us of our salvation and eternal crown. God Almighty is clearly in charge, even in this messed up world. He is absolutely powerful, infinitely wise, a genius, and completely objective. He has no rival on earth, in heaven, or the heavenlies. He is invincible and never changes.

This is the heart of spiritual warfare: God and his truth against Satan and his lies. There is no middle ground. We either belong to God and follow him, or we belong to the world and live under Satan's control (1 John 5:18–19).

How do we fight this enemy? We have been given several pieces of armor (Eph. 6:12–17), two of which are the belt of truth and the sword of the Spirit—the alive Word of God. We cheat ourselves and Satan is delighted when we do not access every verse, every truth, and every promise of our Bibles.

Every verse of Scripture is inspired by God and profitable to us (2 Tim. 3:16–17), so we should not claim verses we like and ignore those that convict us. That's what Satan desires. None of us is so perfect and holy that we gladly welcome every word. Yet, his Word fills us with the power we need to repel the assaults to our soul. There is a specific reason each word was included.

Reflect: If you don't have a Bible reading plan, do not fear—jump right in. Start with the book of John, followed by the other gospel accounts (Matthew, Mark, and Luke). As you fill your mind with the words of God and follow his instruction, you will be able to confront and conquer toxic thoughts and emotions.

Satan's Schemes

Many people ask if a Christian can be possessed by a demon or demons. Because Christ defeated Satan at the cross, believers cannot be possessed by Satan. In other words, a Christian will never belong to the realm of Satan. Demons have no authority over believers. Paul did say Satan can make significant inroads into a believer's life. A person may yield to demonic temptation, accusation, or deception (TAD).

When Satan's schemes, or TAD's, successfully inhibit our heart, mind, and body, we feel emotionally like failures and physically drained. Hope vanishes. Jesus tells us why, "The thief comes only to steal and kill and destroy." Then he said, "I have come that they may have life, and have it to the full" (John 10:10).

Think about this: One day you are sitting in your living room reading a book when a strange man walks in without knocking. He walks over to your television set, picks it up, and then walks out with it. He returns. This time he runs out with your purse. What would you do? Yell, "Wait! You forgot to take my husband"? No. You'd fight back, most likely by calling 911.

Jesus said, referring to Satan and his demons, "How can anyone enter a strong man's house and carry off his possessions unless he first ties up the strong man?" (Matt. 12:29). Satan's power is already broken by Jesus; however, he will not let go of anything he thinks he can control until we exercise the authority and power we have been given through Jesus Christ.

In everyday terms that means he instills fear: fear of failure, of harm, of not being accepted, of anger, and of purposelessness in our lives. Fear begins when we're kids and is carried into adulthood. We become terrified no one will like us or we won't measure up. When we live in this kind of fear, we usually can't hear our Father's voice or sense his presence. It is normal to find a way to calm our fears, so we create a person we believe others will love and accept—the Cover Girl. Then we feel pretty good about ourselves.

Realize Satan is also the perpetrator and propagator of lies. He alone can't destroy things like our marriage or finances. It is his lies and accusations that have the power to destroy. Somehow, evil spirits entice individuals to carry out the depraved desires that surface from their flesh. How does this happen?

First, we give him access. Satan fires that dart and plants the lie in the form of a *potentially* jealous or fearful situation. We listen to the accusation: *You won't get the promotion because she's better than you.* Or, he'll plant a deceptive thought: *Isn't that an attractive man? Don't you want to get to know him better?* He's crafty because he doesn't say, "I'm going to lead you into an affair," even though that is his motive.

Then we think about the lie (or the sin) and dwell on it.

We become preoccupied with the message and then begin to entertain what has been placed in our minds. We've taken a bite of the bait! We contemplate the message feels or sounds right, so we believe the lie. The lie looks attractive and a desire is conceived. We rationalize the lie and then consent and act on it, which gives birth to sin. Our beliefs get stronger that produce toxic emotions (i.e. fear, jealousy, despair, or anger) and sinful behavior (i.e. gossip, an affair, lying). Every adulterous affair was first a fantasy. Every kidnapping was once a thought. Every lie is covered in fear.

Cain and Abel (Gen. 4:1–16) were the first and second sons of Adam and Eve. Cain, a farmer, commits the first murder by killing his brother Abel, a shepherd, after God rejects his sacrifice, but accepts Abel's. God told Cain he would receive his acceptance if he would make the right choice. Instead, he rejected God's acceptance—the ultimate gold key to self-worth. He began to listen to Satan's TAD's and acted on those sinful thoughts.

Abel belonged to God. Cain belonged to the devil (1 John 3:12). Cain's jealous anger drove him to murder Abel. Feeling rejected, he lied to God. Instead of confessing his sin, he said, "Today you are driving me from the land, and I will be hidden from your presence" (Gen. 4:14). Score Satan—relationship broken!

Cain did not master his sin. Instead, sin overtook him and destroyed his life. All we know is Cain went to live east of Eden. Perhaps he became a workaholic, or a rebel, or an alcoholic, or a people-pleaser, searching for that divine acceptance we each crave.

One way we resist and cut off Satan's access is by "testing the spirits to see whether they are from God" (1 John 4:1). We line up that thought or accusation against the Word of God, the voice of truth. The Bible says, "Those who are led by the Spirit of God are sons [*daughters*] of God. For you did not receive a spirit that makes you a slave again to fear, but you received the Spirit of sonship [*adoption*]" (Rom. 8:14–15).

God's spirit touches our spirits and confirms who we really

are: Father and daughter (Rom. 8:16). We are not slaves to fear. This is the voice of truth.

We defend ourselves with prayer, as Jesus and Paul did. We acknowledge a specific area of our life may be empowered or targeted by Satan. In Jesus' name, we send him away directly and out loud (Satan can't read minds). "Satan, in the name of Jesus Christ, I command you get away from me now. I'm Jesus's daughter. You have no power over me. Be gone!"

Each time we wield the words *In the name of Jesus*, we exercise our authority and power over Satan and his demons. You have that power! When God lives in you your body will be as alive as Christ's! (Rom. 8:11).

We need to move beyond knowing we have access to God's power and now actually use it. The power to break that mask comes from our faith and complete dependence on the Lord. The world is not going to change. Satan is not going to change. The people in our lives are not going to change. God made us weak enough so we'd lean on him, enabling us to change.

The Bible says, "Be strong in the Lord and in his mighty power" (Eph. 6:10). We are only as powerful as the measure of our submitted heart. Think of it this way: you have strength stored up in your bicep muscle. It's not until you throw that punch, using the strength in the bicep muscle, that you defer that power.

Paul wrote to the Ephesians, "I pray you will begin to understand how incredibly great his power is to help those who believe him. It is that same mighty power that raised Christ from the dead" (Eph. 1:19–21, TLB). Use that power to R.E.S.I.S.T!

Reflect: Set aside a specific time each day to pray. It is our expression of our trust in God. Present yourself to God either in spoken word or written prayer. Reflect on how you feel as you open up your Bible or devotional book. Often I pray: "Father, I'm feeling tired and easily distracted. Help me to focus on you and your Word. Quiet my mind." Be exactly who you are. It's okay to come before God just as you are—a mess.

Secondly, choose a passage of Scripture to read. One powerful passage is John 17:20–23. Read each verse out loud. Then substitute your name for each word "them" and "they" in verses 21–23. ("Them" and "their" refers to the disciples in verse 21.) Reread the passage. Hear Jesus's voice speaking to you personally. Ask yourself: How am I now relating to God? Am I learning anything about myself? Is God urging me to read further?

The First Devise

Perhaps you've caught reruns of the popular Sci-Fi series *The Twilight Zone.* "You are about to enter another dimension, a dimension not only of sight and sound but of mind. A journey into a wondrous land of imagination. Next stop, the Twilight Zone!"

The Twilight Zone is a self-contained fantasy, science fiction, or horror story often concluding with an eerie or unexpected twist. Perhaps you feel you have just entered the twilight zone ..."a fifth dimension beyond that which is known to man. It is a dimension as vast as space and as timeless as infinity. It is the middle ground between light and shadow, between science and superstition, and it lies between the pit of man's fears and the summit of his knowledge." [35]

When we speak of the supernatural and the invisible, it feels like the twilight zone. However, the Bible is clear this dimension is not of our imagination. It is real. How do we begin to understand all this? Satan's first devise is to present the bait and hide the hook. By this devise, he took our first parents, Adam and Eve.

Let's go back to the very beginning, to Genesis. The central theme in Genesis 1 and 2 is the interrelationship of the Lord God with his creation, Adam. Scripture says, "God said, 'Let us make man in our image, in our likeness'...God saw all that he had made, and it was *very good*" (Gen. 1:26; 31, *my emphasis*). God must have felt deep joy and satisfaction. His plan was complete.

When God said he created man in "*our* image," he was

referring to the Father, Son, and Holy Spirit. God is a relational being. The animals God created have instinctive feelings and needs, but man has a freedom and power that is different than any other species. We have a moral nature, a soul, and the capacity for the spiritual, for love, as well as the ability to think, feel, and make decisions, which is in the image of our Creator.

Unlike other created entities, our brain gives us the ability to make choices that involve changing our environment and ourselves. Creatures can only adapt. Human beings can reason. Our whole person, our soul, is created in God's image.

Then God caused the man to fall into a deep sleep, took one of his ribs and made it into a woman, and brought her to the man. "This is it!" Adam exclaimed (Gen. 2:23, TLB). I love that paraphrase. She must have been a woman of unparalleled beauty. A special gift to Adam, she made his existence complete.

Man and woman were created to have an intimate relationship with God. Given free will, they could choose to love God or not. Every day, man chooses to obey God or disobey him, to take the path of good or of evil, to be blessed or cursed. God's giving us an incentive to choose him. Scripture says, "If you are willing and obedient, you will eat the best from the land" (Isa.1:19). Our reward—an abundant life!

God's plan was never to force himself upon his created. But he had one requirement for Adam and Eve—obey him. One rule is mentioned: "God commanded the man: 'You are free to eat from any tree in the garden; but you must not eat from the tree of the knowledge of good and evil, for when you eat of it you will surely die'" (Gen. 2:16–17). The punishment for eating from this tree was separation from the Father and loss of dominion over creation.

Why would God even give his beloved creatures a tree of good and evil to begin with? It seems as if he wanted to tempt them. God will never tempt us (James 1:13). Is God the author of sin and evil? No. First, God created the world "good." Second, when God created man he gave us free will. For humans to be genuinely free, there has to be an option: obey or disobey God. The tree of the knowledge of good and evil symbolized that choice. God gave Adam the freedom to choose independently—to obey or not.

If God didn't give us a mind of free will, we'd be prisoners or like androids, like the Stepford wives—submissive, beautiful, and zombie-like! It is Satan's nature to tempt us to disobey, not God's nature. The tree of good symbolizes trusting God to tell us what is right or wrong, good or bad. The tree of evil symbolizes trusting our own judgment, making decisions independently from God.

In the next scene, Satan appears to Adam and Eve in the garden as a serpent. Apparently sometime between the completion of creation, which God pronounced "very good," and this point, the fall of Satan occurred. An evil force was present within creation. He did not approach Eve in his true nature; he masqueraded using the serpent.

We've all heard the saying "what a snake" in reference to someone who is deceitful and crafty. The snake is one of the most feared in the animal-reptile kingdom. They move about undetected, and many species kill their prey with one quick, venomous strike. Satan is that snake, a counterfeiter and destroyer.

In the original creation, mankind was extremely significant. Adam was to rule over all the creatures, including the serpent. Adam had dominion in the garden until this particular serpent, Satan, usurped this dominion through temptation and deception. Adam had been given authority, but if, like Lucifer, he rebelled against God, he would lose his power and his perfection. He would become a slave to Satan, to sin, and to God's wrath (Rom. 6:17; Eph. 2:3). Satan's plan was to get Adam to believe his lies, thereby killing man's relationship with God.

Reflect: Mediate on Acts 17:26–28. What is God saying to you in these verses?

The Hinge: Genesis 3

Genesis 3 is said to be the hinge of the Bible. If it were deleted, the key to understanding Scripture in both the Old and New Testaments would have no meaning. It is also a critical piece of narrative about relationship and good and evil. Chapter 2 ended with a short but striking account of the perfection of the first human beings. Chapter 3 opens with an account of their degradation and ruin.

Subtly, the serpent enticed them to eat the forbidden fruit. Satan questioned God's Word. When he says to Eve, "Did God really say you must not eat from any tree in the garden," he was planting seeds of doubt (Gen. 3:1). Recall, God gave Adam the directive because Eve had not been created yet (Gen. 2:17).

First, how did Eve get the command? Did Adam pass the message on to her? If so, maybe he didn't relay it as God spoke it. Or, did God tell her? Did the serpent tell her? The Bible isn't clear if she was even given the command correctly.

Satan impresses on Eve that God has put restrictions on them; therefore, his plan is flawed. Basically, *Rethink what God has said to you. You owe it to yourself!* He says, *God's lying to you! You won't die! God knows when you eat it, you'll become like him!* The serpent now brings into the picture a will other than God's by directly contradicting God's commandments. He tells Eve she'll be as wise as God and won't die if she eats from the forbidden tree.

Satan is questioning God's goodness, *If God really loved you, he wouldn't keep it from you.* This is a lie. He whispers the same lie to children of divorce: "If you were really a good boy, then mom and dad would love each other," or "If your husband really loved you, he wouldn't work on Saturdays." Every person who has lived since then has been tempted with the same words, *Did God really say?* and *God did not really say.* Faith means taking God at his Word.

Satan denies God's Word and substitutes his own lie. This

Kimberly Davidson

was the first deceit of Satan. He tempted Adam and Eve to be like God in a way that God never intended, namely, in self-reliance. *Eve, check it out! This is what God wants for you, for your eyes to be opened liked his!* Adam and Eve were already made in God's image, but Satan tempted them with an even greater privilege—to be like God! Recall, this was his great ambition when he was Lucifer. What he didn't tell them is God never intended them to be like him, to be self-reliant. We were created to be God-reliant.

When Satan said, "Surely you won't die," he lied! Adam and Eve didn't have a sin nature, so Satan appeals to a virtuous desire in Eve. Basically he says, *God wants you to grow up and think for yourself. Use your wisdom. God will reward you for it.* She most likely thought, *Eating from this tree will enhance my spiritual growth. This is a good thing!* The serpent's suggestion appeared true in her judgment. Eve obviously didn't grasp the seriousness of this decision, as we often don't.

Reflect: Tempting our good or virtuous side is usually more powerful than tempting our wicked side. We are more likely to fall to temptation and steal food or clothes for a baby in need, versus sleep with our sister's husband. Eve didn't grasp the seriousness of this decision, as we often don't if we believe the reason is justified.

The World's Greatest Tragedy

The essence of sin is to seek to be independent of God. If Satan can get you to act and think independently of God's will, he can then control your life. You may think you're acting freely, which is part of his deception, but you are actually following what he has placed in your mind and heart. Satan persuaded Adam and Eve that their disobedience would guarantee them an abundant life. They believed him and immediately began to experience sin's consequences.

The story continues, "Then the eyes of both of them were

opened, and they realized they were naked" (Gen. 3:7). Were they blind prior? No. This verse alludes to their being able to see many things they couldn't see before. *Eyes* is translated from the Hebrew word *ayin*, which means *knowledge*.

"Then the man and his wife heard the sound of the LORD God as he was walking in the garden in the cool of the day, and they hid from the LORD God among the trees of the garden" (Gen. 3:8). This verse implies God was with them in human form (like Christ on earth was). At this time, sin did not separate God and mankind. He walked with them in direct fellowship. This is our future hope in eternity (Rev. 21:3).

God called to the man. "Where are you?" (Gen. 3:9). Why would God ask this when "nothing in all creation is hidden from God's sight" (Heb. 4:13; Jer. 23:24)? He was giving him an opportunity to come forth and admit his sin—to confess.

Adam answered God. "I heard you in the garden, and I was afraid [*fear*] because I was naked; so I hid [*shame*]" (Gen. 3:10, *my emphasis*). When we lose our security, fear sets in, so we hide because we feel ashamed and guilty. This is silly because we can't hide from God.

Then God said, "Who told you that you were naked?" Adam knew he had sinned because his eyes were opened. He asked, "Have you eaten from the tree that I commanded you not to eat from?" (Gen. 3:11)

Obviously God knew he ate. He was telling Adam that until he came out from hiding they could not have a relationship. If we were in that garden, we might have heard something like, "Children, stop hiding and running from me. Come here, just as you are. Let's talk. I want a genuine relationship with you."

God was giving Adam another chance to confess, calling him back into relationship. Instead of confessing, he blames God and Eve: "The woman you put here with me–she gave me some fruit from the tree, and I ate it" (Gen. 3:12). When we do wrong, we often try to relieve our guilt or shame by involving someone else. When I was a kid, when I did something wrong, I'd always try to involve my brothers so they'd get in trouble too.

Then God said to the woman, "What is this you have done?"

She said, "The serpent deceived me, and I ate" (Gen. 11–13). Eve recognized she was deceived. Some say she shifted the blame to the serpent, but I see it differently. She confessed and took responsibility for her actions. Adam, on the other hand, felt shame, using fig leaves to cover his nakedness. When he was caught he blamed Eve and God for his mortal decision to eat the fruit.

Eve's words, her confession, broke the bond Satan had over her because eating the fruit was no longer a secret. James counseled, "Therefore confess your sins to each other and pray for each other so that you may be healed" (James 5:16). There is healing power in confession. We all mess up. So, when we blow it, be honest and admit it—confess. It is a process of becoming open, real, and honest with God and ourselves.

Reflect: God is saying to you, "Where are you at today?" Of course he knows. He wants to hear from your heart. He wants a genuine relationship. Stop hiding … stop trying to change on your own … stop running … admit you don't have it all together.

Fess Up

Confession is a major step in changing your mind. Our natural reaction is to hide or minimize our mistake. We only damage our relationships further by erecting walls of stubborn pride, silence, fear, and shame. Any sin we harbor, yet refuse to acknowledge and confess, gives Satan an opening for further attacks. Confession breaks down the walls of brokenness and separation.

Confession is not always easy and once is not enough. The wounds sin inflicts can go deep. Many of us hold secrets. To confess, or "fess up," means we simply agree with God that our behavior is wrong. We sinned. We don't defend our actions. We talk about our feelings and concerns with God, as we would a best friend. Fessing up is always followed by God's instant and complete forgiveness. It clears the obstacles out of the way that could hinder our relationship with him and others.

Both James and Paul counseled that when we sin we not only tell God, but at least one other person (Rom. 10:10). Confessing to another person lets in the light and destroys Satan's grip (John 8:12). Evil hates light because the light of truth destroys deception. We begin to move from brokenness to wholeness. Wholeness is restoration of the spirit, heart, mind, and body.

God always sees us in light of what he intended us to be. He always seeks to restore us to that design. He knows the areas in you that need to be confessed and changed to bring completeness and mind renewal in your life.

What specific areas does God need to change or touch in your life? Be aware, it will be the sting of pride which will discourage you from confessing. But it will be your desire to please God which will compel you to relieve oppressive burdens.

Are you living with unending guilt and shame over something you have done? We're pretty good at piling on shame. "What I did was awful. God could never forgive me." The Bible says the only sins we haven't been forgiven for are the ones we haven't confessed (1 John 1:9). Transforming your sin from unforgivable to forgiven is simply a matter of asking and receiving.

Some Christians think they have committed an unforgivable sin. The only unforgivable sin mentioned in Scripture is blasphemy against the Holy Spirit (Mark 3:29; Matt. 12:31–32). The term blasphemy may be generally defined as *defiant irreverence*. We apply the term to such sins as cursing or slandering God, willfully degrading God, attributing some kind of evil to God, or denying him due glory.

This case of blasphemy, however, is a specific one, called "the blasphemy against the Holy Spirit." It is called the unpardonable sin, and is a willful suppression of the truth about Christ. Continual rejection of the Holy Spirit's promptings to trust in Jesus Christ is blasphemy. It is a hardened, persistent, intentional attitude to reject the Holy Spirit.

Only those who have tuned their backs on God and who willfully deny the truth and have chosen consciously not to affirm what they know to be real need to worry. Whoever rejects the prompting of the Holy Spirit removes him or herself from the only power that can lead her or him to repentance and restoration with God. Pray that you and your loved ones will never suppress God's truth.

The Bible links confession with prayer. Prayer is not designed for us to inform God of our needs or problems because he already knows. Prayer enables us to experience God more intimately. To our surprise, we discover he actually knows what is better for us as our confession unfolds. If we want a powerful prayer life—a great relationship with God—we must regularly confess our sin. Then there are no obstacles separating us from him. We get one step closer to breaking down a nasty mindhold.

Adam, on the other hand, wasn't deceived. In his letter to the Romans, Paul places the primary blame on Adam (Rom. 5:12–21). He felt ashamed and used fig leaves to cover up. When he was caught he blamed Eve and God for his mortal decision to eat the fruit. But in the end, judgment came on all three of them—Adam, Eve, and the serpent.

This was also the beginning of the blame game. We can assume that before the serpent, every conversation was perfectly, completely truthful and honest. All we have to do is take a look around at our conversations today to see the effect of this one moment. Paul Tripp, author of *War of Words*, expressed it well, "No longer do we simply reflect the image of God with our words; we also reflect the image of the serpent. No longer do we consistently speak up to God's standards; we speak down to the serpent's."[36]

Our toxic words can do incredible damage. They can be abusive and tear down one's self esteem. They can cut like a knife into the heart. Used over and over, they may ruin a life by creating deep, damaging mindholds. Words can also do great good. They can make someone feel special and beautiful and valued and loved. They give courage and hope.

That sin was the greatest catastrophe ever. Because of their mistake, we know evil and suffering today. Their sin brought judgment, affliction and death to every person who has ever lived. Theologians call this "the fall." [Some call it the "flaw."]

You ask, "Fallen from what?" Fallen from a relationship with God. The spiritual consequence was death, which in this case means the separation from God. Of course, physical death was the other consequence. Death is not a punishment from God. It is a consequence of sin. For example, some people state they have a "dead" marriage. The reason they have conflict, which feels like death, is because of sin.

The direct presence of God was lost and man's understanding darkened (Eph. 4:18). From that day forward, every baby inherited a sinful nature (called original sin). Each person born strives for independent control over life, suppressing the truth and knowledge of God. [The origin of sin is a mystery. Scripture offers no explanation or cause.]

God had to now speak to matters and problems that were previously not of concern: sin, guilt, shame, depravity and death. A means of reconciliation and redemption had to be provided. The stage was set for Jesus's forthcoming.

The New Testament presents the person and work of Jesus Christ as God's ultimate provision for atonement. "Atonement" is the sacrificial work of Jesus for sinners. In his death on the cross, Christ atoned (made amends or reparation) for the sins of mankind such that God is satisfied. Reconciliation with God has been accomplished!

This is God's character—he provides us a way into his family, and the gift of mercy and grace, in the midst of horrific sin.

Reflect: If we are to think and speak up to God's standards, the work begins in our own heart. What might God be urging you to confess to him and someone else? Read Psalm 32:5. Bring any angry, questionable, and hurtful thoughts to God.

R.E.S.I.S.T. Recap

Recognize you are in conflict every day with a thief who wants to destroy you and your relationships. Use God's Word as a mirror to expose any fear, shame, anxiety, and depression. See it for what it is. Your sin is not always the cause.

Embrace a Bible reading plan, enabling you to fill your mind with truth so you can conquer recurring toxic thoughts and emotions. Embrace the fact you don't have it all together and need God's help.

Submit by setting aside a specific time each day to pray. Present yourself to God. Get into the habit of daily confession. What specific areas does God want to change or touch in your life right now?

Identify & Interrogate—In your daily prayer time, choose a passage of Scripture to read. Ask yourself: How am I relating to God? Am I learning anything new about myself? What am I learning about God?

Set your mind and heart on God, accepting the authority and power to fight, which you have been given through Jesus Christ. Your power to conquer comes from your faith and complete dependence on the Lord and from his Word.

Thank and Praise God for loving you just as you are and earnestly seeking you. Make your praise specific rather than general, and often rather than rare.

Tender Choices

We live in a world obsessed with the elimination of pain. Take a stroll down the medicine aisle the next time you are in the grocery store. One aspirin ad promises relief "when you don't have time for the pain." It's a fact. In a pain-filled world, we do not like to hurt. When we have a headache, we take two aspirin and hope the physical ache ceases.

We also look for cures for our spiritual pain. To avoid the pain of sin, we swallow a pill of deception or denial which diminishes the impact and consequence of sin in our lives. The result: we do not feel the burdensome ache of it.

The result of Adam and Eve's disobedience has been called *the curse*. Adam and Eve were now mere mortals, excluded from living forever. They placed themselves in a rebel position of independence from God, choosing to be their own determiners of what would be significant in life. Self-sovereignty became the driving force. What ensues is man's focus turns inward, not upward, "Let us make a name for ourselves" (Gen. 11:4).

Paradise as Adam and Eve knew was destroyed. Do not despair. You and I, as believers in Jesus Christ, will have "the right to eat from the tree of life, which is in the paradise of God" (Rev. 2:7). Evil will eventually be destroyed, and we will be brought into restored paradise. Everyone will eat from the tree of life and live forever (Rev. 8:17; 21:1–4). Amen!

The moment sin came into the world with Adam and Eve; deception, suffering and evil became an inescapable reality. Sin brought a separation from God that causes pain of many kinds. It gave evil a place in our world. It deceives us. We think wrong is right and right is wrong (Prov. 14:12). For most people the difference between good and evil is pretty obvious. What about the not so obvious sinful thoughts?

There are subtle sins that deceive us into thinking they are not so bad. They are so subtle we commit them without even thinking of them as sin. Anger, for example, can take the form of righteous indignation. Pride, the form of pompous self-congratulation.

I always thought sin only meant breaking the Ten Commandments, like committing murder, adultery, or stealing. But I learned through God's Word, sin also means selfishness, jealousy, anger, greed, lust, gossip, pride—all those little white lies we say to protect the feelings of others, and taking home office supplies from work! And when we rationalize these sins, Satan is victorious.

What can we take away from all of this? First, the serpent is closer than we think. Paul said, "I am afraid that just as Eve was deceived by the serpent's cunning, your minds may somehow be led astray from your sincere and pure devotion to Christ" (2 Cor. 11:3). The devil slinks into our homes, slithers through our offices, slips into our conversations, attempting to deceive us just as he deceived Eve. But he can't do much with a person who is sincerely and purely devoted to Jesus Christ.

Second, never underestimate the destructive power of sin, even the little ones. If a person is inclined toward a particular sin, such as anger, a demon may encourage that attitude. Scripture says sins are like "little foxes that ruin the vineyards" (Song 2:15). Small sins soon lead to more serious ones. What started as a lover's jealous quarrel ends in murder. A lustful look leads to pornography and perhaps adultery. Resentment often results in unrighteous and hateful anger. A well-known Christian teacher said, "There is no sin which I am not capable of committing." You can't establish a truce with sin. You must obliterate it, hence, a battle begins.

Reflect: As the Holy Spirit begins to open the doors of perception which were previously slammed shut; we will discover several emotional responses when we decide to go against what we want to do in order to do what we ought to do. We may feel good because we've scored some God points by obeying his commands. On the other hand, truth be told, we may feel a sense of loss because we feel we've missed out on what we really wanted to do. When we get to this crossroad, we must reckon with the true nature of the kind of person we assume we are. Ouch! Examine yourself and discuss this point.

Denying Self

Like me, I'm sure you have been on more than one diet in your lifetime. One woman said, "I've been on a diet for two weeks, and all I've lost is fourteen days." Then she said, "So I joined a health club and spent about four hundred bucks but haven't lost a pound. Apparently you have to go there."

Have you noticed the first three letters of diet are *die!* Often we hate the word diet or exercise because it means giving up what we like and living an existence similar to John the Baptist, who lived on a steady diet of grasshoppers (Mark 1:6). One reason diets and exercise programs fail is because self-denial is tough.

We are usually willing to sacrifice for success or a smaller dress size, but that's about it. Jesus told his disciples that if anyone desires to follow him they must deny themselves (Matt. 16:24). Denying yourself is not the same as self-denial. We intentionally release our entire self to God. This is submission. Why does God tell us to do this? Does he enjoy watching us squirm and suffer? Of course not. God wants every part of you for himself because he loves you and he knows what is best for you.

The real question is: Are we willing to sacrifice the things that are dear to us, like certain habits, which stand between us and God's will in order to set ourselves apart for him and away from the rest of the world? Paul said if we keep on following our fleshly nature, we are lost and will perish.

As a believer, we are bonded to the Holy Spirit, which means we please God with our submission because we want to, not because we have to. When our mind and heart begin to change, our deepest, truest self doesn't desire to sin. God does not merely command obedience, he gives it. "God will circumcise [*cleanse*] your hearts so that you may love him with all your heart and with all your soul, and live" (Deut. 30:6).

As your mind begins to soak up more truth, God cleanses your heart and you begin to pray as Jesus would pray—with pure and humble motives (John 15:7). You don't pray, *Lord, I pray that I can eat fast food five days a week without increasing my cholesterol and gaining a pound.* A renewed mind doesn't lose the power to sin, merely the desire!

Adam affected mankind by giving each one of us a corrupted nature. But Christ came and gives us an incredible gift. We are transformed into a new creation with a new nature. John said, "You, dear children, are from God and have overcome them [*the world, Satan and the flesh*], because the one who is in you [*Jesus*] is greater than the one who is in the world (1 John 4:4, *my emphasis*). Our faith in Jesus overcomes! Our old thinking identifies with Adam. Our new life is converted and identifies with Jesus. Together we are victorious!

Reflect: You have the ability to stop believing the lie that thinking like God and living a godly life is something uncomfortable, awful and unattainable. *You go girl!*

The Price of Sin

As children become more independent, they exercise their newfound self-rule in many ways. One little girl, when asked by her dad to help her mom, asserted, "You're not the boss of me!" What do you think Dad did, and how do you think their relationship was affected? What about the teenager who in a moment of hormonal anger tells Mom, "I'm going to run away with Brian," or, "I hate you for ruining my life!" If you said these things to God, how would you expect him to react?

With God the issue of harmony comes down to one word: *obedience.* If we obey our parents, we are in harmony with them.

If we don't, we are not. As God's daughter, there is nothing I can do that will change that relationship. God is my heavenly dad by spiritual birth and nothing can change that relationship, just as my earthly dad will always be my father because of a blood relationship.

God is so holy he cannot look at sin, which is why we are counseled to confess our sin and ask for forgiveness. "Sin and the child of God are incompatible. They may occasionally meet; they cannot live together in harmony" (John Stott).[37]

Once God forgives us he hits clear, and we back are in harmony again (Col. 2:14). Since I love my heavenly Father, I don't want to do anything to break that harmony, so I work at not sinning. If I do, I confess my actions, God absolves me, and we move on in the relationship. I am set free! Freedom means I am released from sin and able to glorify and enjoy God.

What might hinder our obedience? Pride. Probably after pride is our motive of not wanting to feel guilty, especially in cases of persistent sin such as pride, bitterness, discontent, criticism, gossip, jealousy. When our consciousnesses are loaded down with guilt, we put ourselves under a burden and sense of condemnation. Score: Satan!

We may also fear what we deem are consequences of disobedience. For example, *If I don't volunteer at the church or tithe, God will punish me.* Or our obedience may be tainted to the other extreme, *I'm going to volunteer in the nursery and tithe so God will bless me.* My desire is to get something from God.

God wants the best for you. That is why he wants your obedience prompted by love instead of a lesser motive. He wants you to enjoy and love him. But we cannot love God if we think we are under his judgment and condemnation.

John Owen stated, "The greatest sorrow and burden you can lay on the Father, the greatest unkindness you can do to him is not to believe that he loves you."[38] Notice, he did not say the greatest sorrow and burden we might lay on the Father is persistent sin.

Reflection: God's Word says, "The Lord is blessing us with peace because of our obedience to him" (2 Chron. 14:7, TLB). What is hindering your obedience today?

Effects of Sin on the Sinner

As we begin to understand more of our own brokenness and sinful rebellion, we begin to understand God's love.   But   be prepared to be humbled as your Cover Girl mask is revealed and broken into pieces.

Jesus explained that the difference between spiritual freedom and bondage is a matter of whether one is a son or a servant. "I tell you the truth, everyone who sins is a slave to sin. A slave has no permanent place in the family, but a son belongs to it forever. If the Son sets you free, you will be free indeed" (John 8:34–36).

Our sin has physical, spiritual, psychological, and relational consequences. How does it enslave us? Let's count the ways:

1. Sin may become a habit or even an addiction.

2. One sin leads to another. Sometimes a larger sin is required to cover up a smaller one. David committed murder to conceal his adultery (2 Sam. 11).

3. We tend to deny, or relabel, our sin so we don t have to acknowledge it. Denying our sin is a way of disposing of the painful consciousness of the wrongdoing.

4. We may admit to our wrongness but decline to take responsibility (like Adam).

5. When we deny sin we live in self-deceit. John Calvin said, "The human heart has so many crannies where vanity hides, so many holes where falsehood lurks; is so decked out with deceiving hypocrisy that it often dupes itself."[39]

6. Sin produces insensitivity as we become less able to respond to the promptings of the Holy Spirit and our own conscience. Paul speaks of those whose minds are darkened as a result of rejecting the truth (Rom. 1:21).

7. Since sin makes one increasingly self-centered and self-seeking, there will inevitably be conflict with others: competition, envy, quarreling, and fighting (James 4:1–2).

8. A major consequence of sin is our inability to empathize with others. We are only able to see and care about our own perspective.

Sin is serious and has far-reaching effects—our relationship with God, with others and ourselves. Accordingly, it requires a cure with just as extensive effects. The cure: Slaves of sin can only be set free through the power of God's Word (John 8:31–32).

We may work hard at trying to cover it up, but God is going to work to expose it at some point so we can deal with it. This means we must continually take those sins that our consciences accuse us of to Jesus. He will cleanse our minds and hearts so we will no longer feel guilty and condemned (Heb. 9:14; 10:2). Then we are free to love God with all our hearts, minds, and souls.

God revealed his solution to our sin: repentance. The need for repentance is emphasized seventy times in the New Testament. Jesus' first public word was "repent!" (Matt. 4:17) The Greek word for *repentance* is *meanoia* which means "change of mind." Looking at sin straight in the face opens the door and is the start to changing my mind and heart.

Right now you may be saying, "I didn't sign up for this. This is too revealing and too much work!" You are right. However, God promises, "I will put my Spirit in you and move you to follow my decrees" (Ezek. 36:27). He gives us the ability to follow his decrees because he knows we can't do it on our own.

Reflect: Even if you struggle with some persistent sin, but you love God, it is more pleasing to him than the person—the slave—who doesn't struggle but is just plain proud. How willing are you to expose areas of sin in your life? What are your fears?

The Freedom of Repentance

Two little boys were playing together one afternoon. Harry, the older and much larger boy, took advantage of his weaker playmate, George, by choosing to play basketball, a game where he would continually win. Frustrated, George withdrew and went to sit out by himself, manfully holding back tears. After a short time, Harry grew tired and called, "Hey, George, come back and play. I'm sorry. I'll play a fair game."

George did not respond to the invitation. Cautiously he asked, "What kind of sorry? The kind where you won't do it ever again?"

If our confession does not come out of a desire for repentance, it is merely admission, not true repentance. Therefore, our mind won't change.

Jesus saw repentance as the point when you change your mind and stop trying to do things your own way. Repentance requires we make a U-turn from denial and discord to truth and submission. We must see a need for change in order for it to work. George wanted to know if Harry would willfully decide to make a personal change.

We may want to pawn off the blame for our actions on those who hurt us, or abused us, or ignored us. *They're the ones with the problems!* God's plan is different. He wants to cleanse our heart and then lather on his brand of amazing grace. It is the ultimate submission of self, but the reward is freedom.

Repentance is an inevitable consequence of becoming a new creature, part of the conversion process that takes place under the convicting power of the Holy Spirit. You must have a change of mind in order to grow. If the Spirit guides you towards God's will and you choose not to take action, a time will come when his voice will be muted. Please be wary of resisting the voice of the Spirit. Without a repentant attitude—a persistent desire to get rid of the negative and toxic—Christian mind change and spiritual maturity is impossible. We will continue to struggle.

Kimberly Davidson

Historically, the repentance process has this two-fold message: *I'm a horrible sinner* (I repent). *It's awesome to be forgiven by God* (I'm forgiven). Stop. Amy said, "I will always be a sinner. I will be that way until I die." That's her mindset. So she keeps messing up, sinning, continuing the cycle of confession, repentance and forgiveness, all along feeling guilty for messing up. That is how she will live because this is her mindset. "I know this is wrong but I just can't help myself" and so she sins. Her mind never changes.

There will always be tension between the flesh and the spirit. What I want to do, I do not do. But what I hate I do (Rom. 7:15; 18). That's life on this earth. I've been forgiven! I learn from it and move on.

Repentance actually saves us from devastating physical consequences. David got it when he wrote, "*When I kept silent, my bones wasted away* through my groaning all day long. For day and night your hand was heavy upon me; *my strength was sapped* as in the heat of summer. *Then I acknowledged my sin to you* and did not cover up my iniquity and you forgave the guilt of my sin" (Ps. 32: 3–5, *my emphasis*).

When we are hiding sin in our heart, our body feels it physically. There cannot be physical or emotional healing without the realization of the gravity of sin and without repentance. Coming to a true knowledge of one's sins, as far as that's possible for us, does lead to deep regret and profound repentance.

To say, "I'm sorry I gossiped about you. I won't do it again" is not enough. A deeper response is called for, one that will root out the source of this sin. "I won't gossip about you anymore because I know I am doing it to make myself look superior. And not only does it hurt you, but it harms my relationship with God."

The Bible teaches we are morally accountable to God for our thoughts and actions. Do not think of this as unfair and ruthless. It spells hope! Hope we can overcome all conflicts and obstacles put in our lives. No matter what we've done, where we've come from, God can give us a better life!

Our relationship with God will never break. We can always

work on the harmony of our relationship. The best way to do that is through prayer, Bible reading, a submitted heart and repentance. "He who conceals his sins does not prosper, but whoever confesses and renounces them finds mercy" (Prov. 28:13).

Reflect: Read Psalm 51. Daily, ask God to reveal what needs to be repented.

The Freedom of Submission

Most of us desire a taste of what life could be if freed from our past and the lies we have believed. Freedom requires falling hopelessly before God which gives us a realistic view of who we are. This doesn't mean you have neurotically low self-esteem. The greater our self-worth, the easier it is to humble ourselves before God. This is called submission.

Repentance requires honest submission. Everything in the world teaches us the opposite, to lead and be independent. "*Submit* yourselves, then, to God. *Resist* the devil, and *he will flee* from you" (James 4:7, *my emphasis*). It's very important that you notice the order in which you are to act—submit first, resist second.

The word *submit* means to line up under another's authority. "When we line up under God's authority we're not alone. Someone is standing beside us who is far mightier than the enemy. Anyone who attempts to fight evil without God is presumptuous, and as they say is "cruising for a bruising."

There are times when you are powerless, or feel powerless, to remove ungodly influences, so you must remove yourself or the source. This might be a person or your computer, whatever is coming between you and God.

Submission is different than surrender, although we use the words synonymously. Surrender is a total relinquishment of control, a declaration of spiritual bankruptcy. *I've hit rock bottom. I can't do this any longer in my strength.* When there are no other perceived options, we surrender in complete dependence on God. Often the total surrender state is not experienced for months or years. What takes place in the absence of surrender is willing submission.

It is human nature to want to take control of our situations. We must be willing to submit to the experience, the expertise, and direction of God and others. It may be the simple act of following directions or obeying one command. Submission is giving my permission to God to work his grace in my life.

Reflect: "Trust in the LORD with all your heart and lean not on your own understanding" (Prov. 3:5). Trust and submission go hand in hand. Do not allow the devil to discourage you from taking the next step. Give God permission to tenderly begin his transformation process.

R.E.S.I.S.T. Recap

Recognize that sin interferes with the harmony of your relationship with God and others. Old thinking identifies with Adam, but your new life is converted and identifies with Jesus. Your deepest, truest self doesn't desire to sin, restoring harmony with God!

Embrace that your sin may be causing you physical problems or to live in denial. Allow God to work to expose it. Embrace the freedom of repentance and the voice of the Spirit. Without a repentant attitude, mind change and spiritual maturity is impossible.

Submit any attitude and/or habit that stands between you and God's will. Begin to work to reject indulging yourself according to the world's rules by submitting daily to the leading of the Spirit.

Identify & Interrogate sinful thoughts, such as being overwhelmed by the power of fear or temptation, or the fire of anger or the pit-y of depression. *Ask God to reveal what needs to be repented of.* Confront that desire or stressor. Repent and conquer it.

Set your mind and heart on God lining up under his authority. Be willing to submit to the experience, the expertise, and direction of God as well as others. What stumbling blocks do you have to doing this?

Thank and Praise God that you can always work on the harmony of your relationship through prayer, Bible reading, a submitted heart, and repentance. Thank him for beginning his amazing transformation process and giving you unlimited chances.

Part Two

Evaluating the Present

"For my thoughts are not your thoughts, neither are your ways my ways," declares the LORD.

–The prophet Isaiah, Isaiah 55:8

A man [*woman*] should take away not only unnecessary acts, but also unnecessary thoughts, for thus superfluous acts will not follow after.

–Roman emperor, Marcus Aurelius Antoninus Augustus[40]

Jesus taught that "the things that come out of the mouth come from the heart, and these make a man [*woman*] 'unclean.' For out of the heart come evil thoughts, murder, adultery, sexual immorality, theft, false testimony, slander ... You are already 'clean' because of the word I have spoken to you."

–Jesus, Matthew 15:18–19; John 15:3

The State of Your Soul

In the fantasy film *Edward Scissorhands,* the character Peg visits a pseudo-medieval mansion on a hill where she finds Edward, a scarred up creation with scissors for hands. She decides to take him home and adopt him into her family.

In a series of flashbacks, we get a glimpse of Edward's creation process. My heart went out to Edward when his creator died, leaving him an orphan (and without human hands). He always looked so sad and incomplete. I couldn't help but flash to Adam and Eve and think the same. Like Edward, they lost the relationship with their Creator. Emptiness found a home in their hearts.

Since the fall, mankind has been cut off from their Creator. Having lost their source of value and belonging, Adam and Eve established insecurity for all of mankind. Life became in the flesh. Man became fearful, anxious, full of shame, guilt, and evil.

Before the fall, Adam and Eve were naked and unashamed (Gen. 2:25). After, they covered themselves, hiding from their Creator. The first toxic emotion was expressed—fear (Gen. 3:10). Nothing opens the door to sin faster than fear, particularly, fear of failure. We can also become comfortable with fear or worry.

We each have two important groups of mindsets: positive faith-based emotions and negative fear-based emotions. Faith and fear are not just emotions, but spiritual forces with chemical and electrical representation that move from the brain throughout the body. They directly impact bodily function.[41] However, there is a difference between the emotion of fear and the spirit of fear. Emotional fear is God-given. Spiritual fear is from Satan.

Positive fear keeps you alive. It motivates you to buy home

insurance (fear of fire), to follow the law (fear of prison), or to obey (fear of discipline). We fear God: "The fear of the LORD is the beginning of knowledge" (Prov. 1:7). To fear the Lord means we hold him in reverence with respect and in awe. Scripture says, "God is greatly feared; he is more awesome than all who surround him" (Ps. 89:7).

Negative emotions evolve out of fear and are from the enemy. Fear stands for: *False Evidence Appearing Real*. Our greatest crises come from a spirit of fear. We're afraid of failing, afraid of being alone or rejected, afraid of running out of money, afraid someone will let us down, afraid that we won't find a husband or a job.

When you live in a constant state of anxiety or fear, most of life passes you by because you are physically, emotionally, relationally, and spiritually unable to focus on anything else. You lose all ability to concentrate and, therefore, are unable to ingest truth. The truth about fear is it is rooted in the belief that God's Word won't work.

Spiritual fear is an awful motivator. It's like a vicious dog chasing us until we are either too exhausted to go on or we get stuck up a tree. Fear attacks your mind: *You are not pleasing to God, Your mom won't love you if you fail, If you don't do this* [...] *then you will be punished.* Worst of all, fear misdirects our thinking to ourselves rather than toward Jesus. It can destroy you.

Nothing should cause you to fear. There is nothing so deeply imbedded in your heart or mind that God's grace cannot reach down and remove it. One woman said God never answered the *whys* of her fear. He pointed her to his personal Word that he, "did not give us a spirit of timidity [*of cowardice and fear*], but [*has given us a spirit*] of power and of love and of calm and well-balanced mind and discipline and self-control" (2 Tim. 1:7, AMP). We are from God, and therefore have overcome any demonic spirits because Jesus, who is in us, is greater than Satan (1 John 4:4). We remind the devil of what God says and stand firm.

Faith, on the other hand, is like a cool breeze on a hot day, refreshing us and giving us the strength to continue on our journey. "Faith is being sure of what we hope for and certain of what we do not see" (Heb. 11:1). It's a gift from God and the essence of our soul. Faith shouts back to fear, using God's Word.

God says, "Fear not, for I have redeemed you; I have summoned you by name; you are mine" (Isa. 43:1). Faith shouts back to Satan, "I am not going to [...] because I'm God's daughter!" There is no area in your life so painful, no offense so heinous, that God's love cannot enable you to break down mindholds of fear, anxiety, or worry.

Reflect: Consider God's track record. God has done all that he has promised.

The writer of Hebrews wrote, "God *can't* break his word. And because his word cannot change, the promise is likewise unchangeable. We who have run for our very lives to God have every reason to grab the promised hope with both hands and never let go. It's an unbreakable spiritual lifeline (Heb. 6:18–19, Msg.)

Fear leaves when you can rely on something that can't fail. There are over one thousand predictions or prophecies in the Bible. None of these promises have failed. Read 1 Kings 8:56 and ask yourself: Do I fear change? Am I willing to allow God do what ever is necessary in order to free me?

Thorny Shame and Pride

We also inherited shame, a cancer of the soul. Shame is the inherent feeling of never measuring up, of pure defectiveness, requiring self-worth to be restored. I experienced over twenty years of being under Satan's thumb of shame, unable to experience the fullness of Christ. This is toxic shame. I felt deeply ashamed of myself. No one did what I did—steal food, eat discarded food, and mess up public toilets. *I was a bad person, like garbage.*

I began to pray, asking God to enable me to identify and confront shameful messages. He began to little by little. I faced

God honestly; I opened my heart and saw myself for who I really was: a daughter of the Most High God. "Guard my life and rescue me; let me not be put to shame, for I take refuge in you" (Ps. 25:20).

We are not the only ones who have carried the burden of shame—our Lord felt it as he hung naked and despised on the cross. But he never lost sight of where he was headed. And he put up with all the torment along the way, scorning its shame. We must keep our eyes set on *Jesus,* who both began and finished this race we're in (Heb. 12:2).

The other deadly emotion we inherited was pride. Pride is a blend of self-absorption with an overestimation of one's abilities or worth. King Solomon said pride ends in a fall, while the opposite of pride, humility, brings honor (Prov. 29:23). C.S. Lewis wrote, "A proud man is always looking down on things and people. As long as you're looking down, you can't see what's above."[42]

Don't mix this up with healthy pride. I am proud to be an American. I take pride in the job my employer has asked me to do. The kind of pride the Bible speaks of is the kind that hinders us from doing what brings glory to God.

Satan was determined to make himself like God. Pride baited Adam and Eve to try to become like God (Gen. 3:5). It was the root of the Pharisees' anger toward Jesus. Jesus gave his disciples the power to cast out demons and perform healing miracles (Matt. 10:8) and authority to minister to people, yet they became self-centered, losing power to do God's work.

How often have you told God what he should do? Pride often means we try to use God to accomplish our own selfish purposes, as if he's our magician or slave. God is to be feared, not treated as an object or force to be used or manipulated. He is an end in himself, not a means to an end.

God will break us of it if we allow him to. On several occasions he has convicted me of other, not so obvious, areas of pride, such as interrupting a conversation to insert my viewpoint. Pride insists you be more interested in hearing me than I in hearing you.

Pride is giving the person in front of me in the checkout line the evil eye for taking so long. *Hey lady, I'm more important than you! Hurry up!* If you are a person who is consistently late, you too, communicate the same message.

God wants to fill us with his Holy Spirit, but when we are proud we are already full of ourselves. There's no room for God. Paul gives us a reality check:

> Don't be so naive and self-confident. You're not exempt. You could fall flat on your face as easily as anyone else. Forget about self-confidence; it's useless. Cultivate God-confidence. No test or temptation that comes your way is beyond the course of what others have had to face. All you need to remember is that God will never let you down; he'll never let you be pushed past your limit; he'll always be there to help you come through it.
>
> 1 Corinthians 10:12–13, Msg

Reflect: God will test us for good. But Satan will tempt us for evil. When I see myself for who I really am, unholy and self-obsessed, I go before God broken. I confess it. I am now free from Satan's grip. What have you learned about yourself (your mindset) in this chapter?

Filling the Void with Relationship Bonds

Have you ever noticed that if you clean out your garage or clear off your kitchen counter, it doesn't take too long before the empty space is filled again. Like sand, take a scoop out, and the surrounding sand swiftly fills the hole. That's the way our soul works. We are all born with a void. People today are searching for something to fill that void, to give their lives value or a boost. Few people are truly content with themselves.

We each have a huge hole inside that craves, yearns, longs, and desires because we are deficient, needy, and dissatisfied. Our tendency is to seek that person or thing or religion or substance to fill us because that hole in our soul needs to be filled.

Many of us allow hatred or evil or prejudice to rush in and fill that hole, wreaking havoc. Too often, we put our hope in the wrong people, who become our god. I did. I became entangled with losers who kept me enslaved to their weaknesses, which meant more rejection and mindholds that cut deeper.

When we're super-glued to another person or situation, we often become depressed. Throwing myself at men didn't make me feel more loved. Trying to please guys by squeezing into a size four didn't work either. Why do so many women get into one abusive relationship after another? Two words: *Poor judgment;* a result of feeling unworthy to be in a relationship with a truly loving man.

My first fiancé stole from me. He not only cheated on me but threw his indiscretions in my face. The other significants chose their own devices of betrayal. Betrayal is an ongoing wound inflicted in relationship. The shame of being taken advantage of by these guys only increased self-hatred and self-doubt, which continued to fuel my addictions.

Most of our difficulties can be traced to relationship. Either we are not connecting with God, or we're having difficulty in relationships with others. This is Satan's dominion. He is the perpetrator of breaking down relationships. He knows a direct attack won't usually work against a genuine Christian, so he'll use more subtle tactics. He'll target our spouse or our kids or our finances. Martin Luther said, "There is no estate to which Satan is more opposed than to marriage."[43] Satan seems to know if he can break down your marriage or turn your child against you, he gets you right in the heart.

Satan is doing quite well. The divorce rate remains high and families continue to suffer. We have slowly become a disconnected and isolated people. It has been said the United States has the highest percentage per capita of lonely people. Neuroscientists say that our use of technology distracts from the human experience of face-to-face contact and has a profound impact on the actual wiring of the brain,[44] which affect our relationships. Have you noticed how many songs are written about being lonely? The Beatles's classic goes, "All the lonely people, where do they all come from ... where do they all belong?"

On the other hand, studies confirm women who are rich in friendships enjoy better physical health, live longer, and are less prone to alcoholism, suicide, and mental illness than those who are lonely and isolated.[45] Research indicates chronic pain can be reduced if one reframes their key relationships. Healthy relationships, nurturing, honest, and supportive friendships and family ties, can ease anxiety that may exacerbate pain.[46]

Reflect on Colossian 2:10: "You have been given fullness in Christ, who is the head over every power and authority." Christ fills our void and alone holds the meaning of life because he is life. He alone is the source of our knowledge and power for fulfilling the abundant life promised each one of us. That deserves our praise!

Living Life as a Branch

Who we are, our true personhood which God created, is achieved only when we are in relationship with God and his people. Life is all about connecting and bonding. That's when we usually learn the deepest truths. Jesus said, "I am the vine; you are the branches. If a man remains in me and I in him, he will bear much fruit; *apart from me you can do nothing*" (John 15:5–6, *my emphasis*).

First Jesus tells us he is truth. Now he is telling us we must be in relationship him. There is nothing more important than making a choice to enter into a relationship with Jesus. He said, "I call you friends because I've let you in on everything I've heard from the Father" (John 15:15, Msg). We find freedom and the answers to life's deepest issues through a bond with God through his Son, Jesus, Truth.

Our basic need is for relationship with God *and* each other in order to be whole. God created each one of us to connect, to understand each other's heart, thoughts and soul. How do we do that? We take the time to talk and listen to one another with respect. We open up our own hearts to others. Conversation is the most intimate human activity (not sex). When I began attending women's Bible studies, I liked learning how each woman coped with pressure, loss, and disappointment. It forced me to look outside myself and also to share what was on my heart and mind.

It's not uncommon to use the excuse that we are too busy in order to insulate ourselves from connection. Failure to connect is disastrous for our well-being. Relationships are built by ongoing communication. They cause long-term changes in our brain, which include memories of the relationship and expectations for its future. These changes result in an emotional bond between the two communicating parties.

Bonding with our mother (or other person) during our first year on earth determines how secure or insecure we will be in relationship. Our brain processes that first attachment which is set for life. Most babies bond with their parents. If a baby doesn't bond, it doesn't mean that parent was bad. Perhaps that parent was absent, emotionally or physically, because of illness or a death. Or perhaps the baby could not bond because of infirmity. Each deserves grace.

Ask yourself: "What did Mom (or other person) do to bond with me?" "Whenever there is a major deficit in parental love, the child will, in all likelihood respond to that deficit by assuming itself to be the cause of the deficit, thereby developing an unrealistically negative self-image" (M. Scott Peck, M.D.)[47] If Mom does not bond with me, then as I maneuver through life, I may begin a search for faulty substitutes such as drugs, alcohol, food, or sex, which substitute for the specific losses in relationships.

We may also develop bonds with some teachers, or mentors, or bosses. It is possible that one party develops a stronger bond than the other and ends up getting hurt. Lack of bonding and depression are often related.

If a person to whom we have a special bond dies or wants to break up with us, we experience a sudden, severe emotional pain. When this bond is broken, the activity of the deep limbic system (the part of the brain that controls the automatic systems of the body, our emotions and survival responses) is disrupted, and the pain centers are activated.[48] Many who experience grief say the pain actually feels, literally, like their heart is broken. They may become physically ill.

For some of us, healing requires acknowledging and working through the grieving process—denial, anger, bargaining, depression, and finally acceptance. If you need to grieve a certain loss or losses, I encourage you to talk with a pastor or counselor and locate some good grief resources. Don't try to jump right to the acceptance stage.

Whenever we enter into a relationship with someone, either through choice or through necessity, we create some kind of bond. Our soul becomes tied to this person. We share deep thoughts, dreams, and feelings with each other without fear of rejection. This is the freedom of grace and truth.

Each person has an inner longing only Jesus can satisfy. We can't be filled with Jesus if we are filling ourselves with self, men, or idols. Part of my healing process was recognizing these relationships failed because they were never built on true emotional intimacy. The foundation was only physical. These guys didn't have the answer. God did.

When relationships and the things you see start to fall apart, the things you can't see hold you together. God will meet all your needs (Phil. 4:19). The best thing we can do after coming out of a damaging relationship is take time to be alone with God. The one who longs for God with all her heart will find him (Jer. 29:13). Let him nurse your wounds and begin to cut those invisible bonds. Band-Aids don't work. Only the deep love of Christ will break up the scars and mindholds.

Reflect: List each relationship bond you have today. Label it a P for positive, and N for negative. Which do you have more of: Ps or Ns? If you don't have any meaningful relationships, pray. Ask God to help you identify your specific needs or void and to begin the process of connecting with one person.

Is It Well with Your Soul?

William Shakespeare said, "The brain is the soul's fragile dwelling place." Shakespeare was inferring that our personhood resides in our brain. Biblically, *soul* (the Hebrew word *nepesh*) means "living individual," the whole person, a life. Contrary to popular thinking, we *are* souls versus *have* souls. Our brain speaks to our heart, our mind, and our body—our soul. A healthy brain, therefore, is essential to a healthy soul.

Daniel G. Amen, M.D., neuropsychiatrist and pioneer in the field of brain imaging, states:

> Your brain is the hardware of your soul. It is the hardware of your very essence as a human being. You cannot be who you really want to be unless your brain works right. How your brain works determines how happy you are. How effective you feel, and how well you interact with others. If you are anxious, depressed, obsessive-compulsive, prone to anger, or easily distracted, you probably believe these problems are "all in your head."[49] A healthy soul actually enhances brain function, and a healthy brain is essential to a healthy soul. The brain-soul connection is involved in everything we do.[50]

The psalmist cries, "Why are you downcast, O my soul?" (Ps. 42:11). Our soul agonizes and may even be damaged in some way. Something is missing—the need to belong to God and connect with other human beings. As a baby, that need is usually met in the family unit, but if that unit is dysfunctional, that baby grows up experiencing a damaged soul.

For example: If Mom routinely hits Baby, Baby learns not

to feel in her emotional heart. Her soul is damaged at an early age. Child abuse damages a soul. That child can't love through her soul because she has chosen to abandon a sense of feeling alive. It's her way of living free of pain. *But*, God can love her through her soul.

Dr. Dan Allender wrote, "A victim may choose to kill part of her soul that feels pain, but the grace of God renders her unable to utterly destroy her own or anyone else's intuitive sense of being. She cannot entirely wipe out the pain ... Despair is a protective blanket that shields the soul against the cold demands of harsh self-doubt."[51]

We have to cry out to God and fight for our soul, placing it under the protection of Jesus because Satan won't quit. The power to destroy our soul is not within the control of Satan and is not even within the authority of another human being. Jesus said, "Don't be afraid of these who want to murder you. They can only kill the body; they have no power over your souls" (Luke 12:4, TLB). Because of the way we're designed, it is possible to deaden our soul, but it is also possible to resurrect.

Jesus said a relationship with him brings rest to our souls (Matt. 11:28–29). There is an emotional exhaustion that comes from carrying heavy burdens. You can go on vacation, but your soul won't be restored. It can only be rectified by finding rest in Christ. Jesus spent most of his earthly time surrounded by needy people. He faced relentless opposition. The psalmist cried, "My soul is weary with sorrow ..." The psalmist's answer, "Strengthen me according to your word" (Ps. 119:28).

If there was ever a person who exemplified the right mindset (a mind set on Christ) during a time of trial, it was Horatio G. Spafford. A Chicago businessman, he suffered financial disaster in the Great Chicago Fire of 1871. At the same time, he and his wife were grieving over the death of their son. He realized they needed to get away for a vacation. Spafford booked passage to England. His wife and four daughters went ahead on the ship SS Ville du Havre. He planned to follow in a few days.

While on the Atlantic Ocean, the ship was struck by an iron sailing vessel and sank within twelve minutes. Two hundred and twenty-six lives were lost, including Spafford's four daughters. When the survivors were brought to shore, Mrs. Spafford cabled her husband: "Saved alone." Spafford booked passage on the next ship. As they were crossing the Atlantic, the captain pointed out the place where he thought the SS Ville du Havre had gone down. That night, Spafford penned the words that became a great hymn: "When sorrows like sea billows roll…it is well, it is well with my soul."

In his angst, his psyche was going to be fine. He rejoiced in God. It's going to be okay because my foundation is strong, because my spirit is connected to God.

"Praise the LORD, O my soul" (Ps. 103:22). While we can expect to suffer on earth, Satan cannot harm our soul or take away eternal life with Jesus. As difficult as your situation may be, we can choose to praise God. Practice praise. It breaks the cycle of negative thinking and whining. Find some people that incorporate praise into their lives. They are usually the ones shining! When you find them, take notes.

Reflect: If you are weary, your soul deadened, go to Jesus. Stop. Quiet yourself. Now pray—talk to Jesus, with all your heart, mind, and soul. Prayer is about a relationship with God. That's our first challenge to mind change. It's tough because most of us have provisional prayer (*I want…*) deeply imbedded in our thinking. I'm always working at relational prayer. Praise God for who he is and what he is doing.

Heart Attacks

The Wizard of Oz is a story of a little girl, Dorothy Gale of Kansas, with the help of her friends, who bring down a big, bad witch. It is a story of good against evil.

One of her friends was the Tin Man, who desired a heart. After oiling all his joints, Dorothy says, "Well, you're perfect now." The Tin Man says, "Perfect? Bang on my chest if you think I'm perfect. It's empty. The tinsmith forgot to give me a heart.

All hollow." He breaks out in song: "If I only had a heart, I'd be tender; I'd be gentle, and awful sentimental, regarding love and art. [Oh ...] Just to register emotion, jealousy, devotion, and really feel the part." He follows Dorothy to the Emerald City to get a heart from the Wizard of Oz so he could love and feel emotion again.

Although fiction, we see similarities: the devil versus mankind. The prize: our heart. We perceive our heart is emotion-based versus our mind, which is reason-based. Our anatomical heart is a muscle that works ceaselessly, beating one hundred thousand times a day, clocking up three billion heartbeats over an average lifetime. It keeps the body freshly supplied with oxygen and nutrients while clearing away harmful waste.

Most often we think of our heart as the seat of emotions. Physiologically, our brain is actually the seat of emotion because it manages our entire bodies. It houses areas responsible for memories, thinking, and emotion, as well as speaking and hearing. All of our emotions are a reflection of neurological activity located in the brain, which results in physical responses throughout the body. The mind is what the brain does.[52] It follows, Satan wants our mind.

There is a strong connection between both the heart and mind because our heart is the hub of our entire personality. The Bible likens our heart as the center of our intellectual and rational functions, the things we usually ascribe to the mind. The root of all decisions is the heart (Luke 6:43–45).

The heart is a metaphor for who we are as a person. If I say, "She's got a good heart," I'm not saying her muscular organ is pumping blood through the blood vessels via repeated, rhythmic contractions. I'm saying she is a thoughtful, nice, generous person. It refers to the deepest level of a person and is the source of our deepest wishes and desires (Gen. 6:6; Ps. 14:1; 21:2). *Scripture also says,* "The heart is deceitful above all things and beyond cure. Who can understand it?" (Jer. 17:9)

I'm sure you know a person you'd call a "know-it-all." This person helps everyone else understand where *they* have gone wrong in their thinking. Usually, these people have limited relationships because they are afraid of ever being wrong. The narrow-minded way a "know-it-all" approaches people has more to do with what she's feeling in her heart than what she knows is true in her head.

Jesus said, "Are your hearts hardened? Do you have eyes but fail to see, and ears but fail to hear?" (Mark 8:17–18) A person who is said to have a hardened heart is one whose mind or attitude is dead toward God and even people. They refuse to repent and believe in the promises of God (Ps. 95:8; Heb. 3:8).

As a child of God we are promised a new heart and a new spirit. "I will remove from you your heart of stone [*a hardened heart dead toward God*] and give you a heart of flesh [*a soft, tender, emotion-based heart, able to receive and act upon the truths of God's Word*]" (Ezek. 11:19; 36:26, *my emphasis*).

Reflect: What is the state of your heart today?

A Jolly Heart

It's been said the most wasted day is that in which we have not laughed. Did you know having a good laugh actually strengthens relationship bonds and makes for a stronger heart? Laughter, like water, flushes toxins out of our body. When we laugh, we have the ability to diffuse the pain by physically increasing the body's production of endorphins, the body's natural painkillers.

We need to laugh more. A jolly heart is the human gift for not only a healthy heart, but for coping and survival. It breaks the ice, lowers blood pressure, reduces your risk of developing heart disease, and improves mood. Someone who laughs, particularly at herself, can never take herself too seriously. It's the certain cure for arrogance.

We are responsible for our heart's care. A study found that just fifteen minutes of watching a funny movie *increased* average blood flow by 22 percent while watching a serious drama *decreased* blood flow by 35 percent. Fifteen minutes of laughter and thirty minutes of exercise three times a week is good for the vascular system.[53]

The Holy Spirit, our agent of change, refines and purifies our new hearts, metaphorically speaking, to be more like Jesus's—a person who is full of love, compassion, and emotion. He is pulsating and alive within us, the driving force of changed behavior. It is no surprise King Solomon advised, *"Above all else, guard your heart* [or *affections*] *for it is the wellspring of life"* (Prov. 4:23, *my emphasis*). This is serious. Impossible? God never tells us to do something we can't do in his strength (Phil. 4:13).

Reflect: "Almighty God, create in us a clean heart and renew a right spirit within us, that amid the din and confusion of this noisy world we may always choose the more excellent way. Through Christ. Amen" (Rueben P. Job). [54]

The Receptive Heart

Jesus was a storyteller, his speech filled with parables and images intended to teach his listeners spiritual truth by comparing something familiar with something unfamiliar. Jesus knows that when our brains process word pictures it helps us understand spiritual truth better. In the parable of the sower, Jesus knew most of the people would never produce fruit from changed lives because the Word he was teaching them was like seed falling into poor soil (read Mark 4: 1–13).

The parable tells of seeds that were erratically scattered, some falling on the road and consequently eaten by birds, some falling on rock and consequently unable to take root, and some falling on thorns, which choked the seed and the worms ate them. According to the parable, only the seeds that fell on good soil germinated producing a crop thirty, sixty, or even a hundredfold of what had been sown.

The seed represents God's Word (Luke 8:11). The sower is us, empowered by the Holy Spirit to sow God's Word. The soil is the human heart. Our heart must be prepared to receive the seed before it can take root and produce a harvest.

Let's continue on with Jesus' parable, Mark 4:14–20:

> The farmer sows the word. Some people are like seed along the path, where the word is sown. As soon as they hear it, Satan comes and takes away the word that was sown in them. Others, like seed sown on rocky places, hear the word and at once receive it with joy. But since they have no root, they last only a short time. When trouble or persecution comes because of the word, they quickly fall away. Still others, like seed sown among thorns, hear the word; but the worries of this life, the deceitfulness of wealth and the desires for other things come in and choke the word, making it unfruitful. Others, like seed sown on good soil, hear the word, accept it, and produce a crop—thirty, sixty or even a hundred times what was sown.

In that day, as today, there are four kinds of hearts that respond to God's Word:

One, the hard heart (Mark 4:4, 15), which resists the Word of God and makes it easy for Satan (the birds) to snatch it away. If we recklessly open our hearts to the wrong influences, we are in danger of developing a hard heart (see Prov. 4:23).

Two, the shallow heart (Mark 4:5–6; 16–17). Since there is no depth, whatever is planted cannot sustain because it has no roots. This is the emotional hearer who joyfully accepts God's Word, but really doesn't understand the price that must be paid to become a genuine follower of Christ. She has little or no foundation.

Three, the crowed heart (Mark 4: 7, 18–19). This person receives the Word but does not truly repent and remove the weeds, or sin, out of her heart. Weeds represent worldly desires like wealth, control, or a lust for things. The good seed has nowhere to grow.

Four, the fruitful heart (Mark 4: 8, 20). This is our desire and what we are working toward. When Jesus takes up residence in our hearts, our thinking and actions are naturally impacted. We are truly taking each thought captive to Jesus (2 Cor. 10:5). We become image bearers because fruit—a changed life—is evidenced. The other three kinds of hearts produce no fruit and represent toxic thoughts and emotions.

Reflect: What is the state of your heart? Where are the seeds falling in your life? What is the solution? State two new things you can do to change this status.

R.E.S.I.S.T. Recap

Recognize you were born with a void that must be filled. Your flesh, the world, and Satan is looking to fill it, but only God has the ability to seal any empty space with his grace and mercy. Jesus is our model for creating fulfilling relationships.

Embrace healthy and nurturing relationships. After coming out of a bad relationship, take time to be alone with and embrace God.

Submit to a relationship with God through his Son, Jesus, bringing rest to your soul. God created you to connect and to understand another's heart, thoughts, and soul. Submission is to take the time to talk and listen to one another with respect.

Identify & Interrogate where you may be isolating yourself and who you have special bonds with. What is the state of your heart? Are you willing to share deep thoughts, dreams, and feelings with someone else without the fear of rejection?

Set your mind and heart on God who, for you, has defeated shame, fear, guilt, and pride. Look up. He will never let you down or be pushed past your limit. He'll always be there to help you through.

Thank and Praise God that he did not give you a spirit of fear, but a spirit of power and of love. Praise him for the capability to laugh a lot!

Making Sense of the Mind and Brain

In the *Wizard of Oz*, Dorothy and the Tin Man are joined on their adventure by the Scarecrow, who desires a brain. The Tin Man's desire for a heart notably contrasts with the Scarecrow's desire for a brain or a mind, reflecting a common debate between the relative importance of the mind and the emotions. This, indeed, occasions a philosophical debate between the two friends as to why their own choices are superior; neither convinces the other. Dorothy, listening, is unable to decide which one is right. What do you think? Which is more important: your heart or mind?

The encyclopedia states the *mind* collectively refers to the aspects of intellect and consciousness manifested as combinations of thought, perception, memory, emotion, will, and imagination. It includes all of the brain's conscious processes.55

The Apostle Paul, like many ancient Greek philosophers, thought of the mind as something that has the ability to understand, to reason, and to think (1 Cor. 14:14–19). A human's actions come from the inclinations of his or her mind. Theologian Gregory "the Great" (AD 361) believed the image of God is found in our mind and soul.

Scripture describes the inclination of a person's mind as being either Spirit filled, or controlled by Satan. "The god of this age [*Satan*] has blinded the minds of unbelievers, so that they cannot see the light of the gospel of the glory of Christ, who is the image of God" (2 Cor. 4:4). This is why we have friends and loved ones who seem unreceptive to our testimony and resistant to the Bible.

The Lord can open people's minds. The prophet Isaiah predicted he would come "as a light to the Gentiles, to open blind eyes, to bring out prisoners from the prison, those who sit in darkness from the prison house" (Isa. 42:6–7). Jesus opened the minds of the disciples who walked the Emmaus road with him so they could understand the Scriptures (Luke 24:45).

Some neuroscientists suspect everything that makes people human is no more than an interaction of chemicals and electricity inside the labyrinthine folds of the brain.56 This conflicts with our beliefs and faith. Our brain and our life are inseparably linked.

How we live our life matters. Dr. Daniel Amen states in his book *Healing the Hardware of the Soul:* "The condition of our soul and the spiritual connections we make have a strong impact on the physiology of the brain. It is a reciprocal relationship. I have seen that sin (doing things that you know are wrong) disrupts healthy brain function and leads to anxiety, fear, and depression, while living with integrity and having a positive relationship with God and others actually improves brain function."[57]

Reflect: How can you apply this knowledge to your daily life?

***

Who Are You Today?

It's been stated by some scientists that whether a person is good or evil depends on their state of the mind. We might even say it depends on the state of their heart.

Who we are today is a result of what we've been thinking and believing all our life—our mindset. Our thoughts influence our relationships even though we equate relationships with the heart. One thing I've learned is when we are alone and we take off our mask, then the real person comes out. In André Malroux's *The Walnut Trees of Altenberg,* Walter said, "Essentially a man is what he hides." His father answered sharply, "A man is what he doest."[58]

One of Satan's subtle deceptions is that you can do things

in secret that will never be revealed; for if you reveal your sin or your heartache, you will be rejected or condemned or ridiculed. The fact is we hide what we do. Jesus said, "For there is nothing hidden that will not be disclosed, and nothing concealed that will not be known or brought out into the open" (Luke 8:17). We may successfully hide our secrets from others, but God sees everything we do, things we are accountable for.

We have been sold out by the world and Satan on our weaknesses. Forget about your weaknesses! What about that which is good, the strengths and gifts and talents God gave you? Thomas Edison said, "If we did all the things we are capable of doing, we would literally astound ourselves."[59]

I think one reason we shy away from our strengths is fear. We may have to get involved with life, with the church, and that is risky. We know how much it hurts to be rejected and judged by other people for our past, criticized for our best efforts, or laughed at when we are sincere.

It's easy and safe to stay as we are. We adjust, although we aren't really happy. We feel safe. "Safe" in this case equals darkness. Scripture demands we expose the deeds of darkness as we become aware of them (Eph. 5:11), which is the focus of this journey. I have learned that I'm my best self when I'm living in the light. My best self equates to developing my relationship with God. It also enhances my brain function.

Reflect: How we think, feel, act, and how well we get along with other people has to do with the moment-by-moment functioning of our brain. When our brain works right, we work right. When our brain is troubled, we are weak and a target for Satan.

Prefrontal Cortex

As a minister who counsels women and young girls about mind change, I find brain function and imaging technology fascinating, cutting edge, and very helpful to understanding how we develop and ultimately conquer certain mindsets. Our brain has four main lobes. One of these is the frontal lobe or prefrontal cortex (PFC). The basic activity of this brain region is considered to be an orchestration of thoughts and actions in accordance with internal goals.

When the PFC is working right, we are empathetic, compassionate, and able to express our feelings. We are goal directed and organized. Our conscious (free will and sense of morality) is located in the PFC. It prevents us from impulsiveness, sin, and bad thoughts. If the PFC is not functioning right, we are more likely to say something we may regret later, or do or say something which inflames a situation. If you have a healthy PFC, you learn from your mistakes and move on. You are less likely to make that mistake again—like fall into that particular hole of temptation.

The PFC helps us focus on important information while tossing out less significant or toxic data. When we need to focus on something important, the PFC decreases, distracting input from the other brain areas by inhibiting or filtering that data out.[60] God has designed in each one of us a built-in mechanism to repel the devil's attempts to distract us from important tasks such as prayer, meditation, and developing relationships.

Mark Twain said, "Always do right. This will gratify some people, and astonish the rest." However, we may not be unable to do what is right! Dr. Amen wrote:

> Without proper PFC function, impulses take over, making it difficult to act in consistent, thoughtful ways. Impulse control issues are one of the main components of sin, doing something that you know is wrong. Without full functioning of the PFC, people tend to act on the moment, without forethought or regard for consequences. When the PFC works properly, you have a good sense of right and wrong and you are able to match your behavior to your moral beliefs. You know what you want in life and are able to stay focused. You are able to fully exercise free will.[61]

Kimberly Davidson

Reflect: How does understanding the biology of your brain help you understand yourself better? Your kids? Your spouse? Your parents? In-laws?

The Temporal Lobes

The temporal lobes add emotional spice to life. Often called the *emotional brain,* they house our passions, desires, sense of spirituality, and pleasure. They either give us purpose for living or take us to the pit of depression. They also play an essential role in our personality development.

When both the temporal lobes and limbic system work right, our emotions are even-keeled. We have access to spiritual experiences and control over our temper. When this part of the brain is overactive, negativity can take over. A person with severe decreased activity in her right temporal lobe may worry about or see things that others don't see or hear.[62]

The total experience of our emotional memories is, in part, responsible for the emotional tone of our thoughts and feelings. When these two systems function properly, a person is more up and able to connect with other people. When the limbic doesn't work well, we end up stuck, stagnant, isolated, and feeling disconnected from God. When our attention gets stuck on toxic negative thoughts, or painful memories, or anger, our emotional or spiritual growth comes to a halt. When these parts work right, we are able to be flexible, forgive, and open our minds to growth.[63]

We can conclude then, if our brain isn't working right, we can't be our real selves. However, understanding *the why* of our brain function brings us certain peace about our real selves. Audrey describes her darkest place—coping with chronic depression:

> I began my own research. I found a video which showed how our brain is affected by depression. A list of symp-

toms matched nearly every behavioral change I'd seen in myself. I stopped regarding depression as a horrible curse and looked at it more like diabetes or a health condition requiring treatment. Prayer helped a lot, but I started to view counseling and antidepressants as God's chosen restoration tools. I'm not a freak!

Scientists who have been following families with a history of depression have found structural differences in family members' brains—specifically, a significant thinning of the right cortex, which may be a trait or marker of vulnerability to depression.[64]

In his book, *Change Your Brain, Change Your Life,* Dr. Amen introduces us to a former patient, Sally. Sally was admitted to the hospital suicidal, depressed, and anxious. He discovered she also had many Attention Deficit Disorder (ADD) symptoms and ordered a brain study called SPECT, Single Photon Emission Computed Tomography. Brain SPECT imaging gives a visual picture of brain function by creating a colored picture representing blood flow or chemical reactions in different areas of the brain. Areas of low blood flow show up as apparent "holes."[65]

[A SPECT is a diagnostic tool and is never the final answer. Some insurers and physicians consider SPECT experimental and investigational. It should be used with a good medical history.]

Up to now, Sally had considered herself an underachiever, so much so she contemplated suicide. Her teachers and family possibly reinforced her negative thinking. Sally's brain studies were abnormal, but her response was one of elation! Seeing the SPECT images of her brain was very powerful. She said, "Having ADD is not my fault. It's a medical problem, just like someone who needs glasses."

Audrey and Sally could see their problems weren't all in their heads. These were burdens they need not carry. Knowing what we know about our personal battles, I would guess the enemy didn't allow either of them let those mindholds go so easily. I presume they still had work to do to change their thinking on a permanent basis.

If we protect our brain, we enhance our ability to love, work, and learn, and we are less vulnerable to outside attacks. Our mind needs to be exercised just as our physical body does. The medical community feels that viewing a lot of television has serious health risks because it is passive and sedentary. A TV watcher is not firing many synapses in the brain. A functional MRI scan study showed a difference in brain activity between watching TV and playing board games and participating in robust discussions. The latter activities showed the brain continuing to develop while TV watchers barely registered a blip on the scan study.[66]

Reflect: Boredom is the brain's cry for activity. Scientists agree that keeping our minds active by doing a variety of mental exercises can improve memory, reasoning, and speed of thinking. It is important to learn to do new things. Learn a foreign language or how to play a musical instrument—even driving a new route to work can wake up sleepy brain cells. Tennis and ping-pong are one of the best brain plus body exercises for you!

The Sting of a Thought Dart

Now we can understand why Satan targets our minds. Paul told the Ephesians to take up the shield of faith in order to extinguish all the flaming arrows of the evil one (Eph. 6:16). The flaming arrows are aimed right at our mind. Another term is fiery darts, symbolic of fiery trials or temptations; of distractions or storms; or toxic, evil thoughts. I call them *thought darts.* No matter where our faith level is at, we've all felt the sting of a thought dart that suddenly strikes our mind out of nowhere.

Many ask how Satan does this. Can he read our minds? We know God knows our thoughts (Luke 11: 17), but there is nothing in the Bible to indicate that Satan is omniscient or that he can read our thoughts. The Bible never says demons or angels are all-knowing. Satan is adept at predicting human behavior.

He can predict what you may do in a given situation without knowing your thoughts because of his knowledge of mankind.

Satan discourages us emotionally, spiritually, physically, and financially—any way he can. Today, many of us feel the battle wounds from those thought darts. After a dart hits, our body reacts. The human body is loaded with many different kinds of chemicals and hormones released by our brain in response to our thoughts. Whenever you think awful, miserable, negative thoughts, your brain works less efficiently and is likely to put you into an emotional slump.[67]

Let's dissect the anatomy of a thought: You have a thought. Your brain releases chemicals which can be emotionally toxic or not. An electrical transmission goes across your brain. You become aware of what you're thinking. Thoughts stimulate emotions that result in an attitude which finally produces behavior.

All behavior starts with that one thought. Therefore, negative or toxic thoughts produce toxic feelings, producing toxic attitudes, resulting in noxious behavior. Research shows that approximately *87% of illnesses can be attributed to our thought life,* while only 13% to diet, genetics and environment.[68]

The intent of Satan is to plant a suggestion snowball, which grows in size until you become immobilized. Guilt and rejection are good examples. Satan somehow plants a suggestion in the form of a temptation, an accusation, a lie, or the urge to sin. *You'll never be able to do that. You've failed miserably in the past. They'll just laugh at you.* If I believe this lie, I give up on my task and start a pity-party, bringing my entire family down with me.

Pit-y is emotional quick (or pit) sand! If we fail to resist the fiery darts, the flames of Satan's thought attacks go through our minds, resulting in toxic or sinful behavior. That sin may become greater and greater, such as the snowballing effect of a lie. It becomes so big that it covers the face of God, hiding his grace and love. By establishing defeat, shame, or fear in our minds, Satan can render us ineffective.

When we are in fellowship and intimacy with God, it is *generally* difficult for Satan to attack our spirit. Solomon said a man's spirit sustains him in sickness, but a crushed spirit who can bear (Prov. 18:14)? If our spirit is in good condition, if our relationship and fellowship with God is good, we can keep going, even through physical assaults.

Laura Wilkinson is a diver from Texas who practiced hard for the 2000 Olympics in Sydney. During her training, she broke three bones in her foot. No doubt Satan hit Laura with lies such as: *Too bad, Laura. All that work for nothing. That should make you angry!* Laura could have had a pity party over her lost dream. Instead she chose not to give up. Unable to work out, Laura used mental or guided imagery to practice her dive. She visualized herself climbing up to the ten-meter platform and then walking through the motions of her complex high dives. She envisioned each split second of her approach, posture, position, dive, entry into the water, and swim to the side of the pool.

Her cast came off just before the Sydney Games. She went on to compete and to win the first Gold Medal for a female American platform diver in nearly forty years. Our minds are powerful. We can use them to adjust our attitudes and actions. As we meditate on God's Word, thinking over verses and words day and night, our thoughts become transformed.

Reflect: You, too, can aim to persevere as Laura did through mental imagery. Focus your mind on something specific such as breathing or repeating a word, such as *Father* or *Jesus.* Or select Scripture to quiet your mind. Visualize a positive outcome or scenario.

Are You Perpetuating Toxic Thinking?

When a negative thought pops into your mind, how do you usually respond?

1. What toxic thought?
2. I feel so guilty or ashamed.
3. It's not my fault. The devil made me do it.

Surely you have noticed how you tend to stay upset once hit with that worry, anger, or fear dart. We perpetuate the downward spiral by replaying that thought over and over again. This is a function of the mind.

Every thought carries a "spiritual charge" that moves us a little closer to or a little farther from God.[69] Our thinking processes are a powerful medium, which is why Satan's motive is to attack our thoughts.

The first television interview I did, I made a mistake. Surely laughing, Satan fired that thought dart: *I can't believe you said Jesus said that when it was Paul. You idiot!*

I even answered him, "I know it was Paul. Why did I say it was Jesus? You're right. I'm so stupid."

After wallowing in self-condemnation for a while, I looked up. *Why, Lord, did I mess up that way? Why did you let me say that? I was prayed up!* I felt God whisper, *Don't worry about it!* He reminded me he had arranged the interview. Jesus died for me because I'm not perfect, therefore I didn't have to tape the perfect interview. Plus, no one else was going to have the same reaction I had. Satan just wanted me to think they would.

God gave me a huge dose of grace, and I was off my own hook. But I replayed that mistake over and over in my mind. I allowed Satan to put me back on my own hook repeatedly. *Some so-called expert you are! What will people think of you now?*

I had to take these thoughts captive and work to change my thinking:

1. I recognize this voice is not of God but of Satan. Reject!

2. I get off the road of self-condemnation. Repent!

3. I toss out Satan's message and replace it with God's.

4. I give myself grace and say, "God set up this interview and accepts it as is. He accepts me just the way I am. He knew what he was getting when he sent me. If God accepts me, mistakes and all, I accept me! Move on!"

5. Satan's power is broken.

Some of us allow the world to fill our minds with "stinking

thinking." Some of us are pessimists, drawn to everything negative. Others feel inferior in a crowd of one! Some of us don't even have an opinion.

If I have just described you, imagine Satan and his demons cheering! How do we fight back? We use our mind. We mull over things that are truthful and pure—things that steer us often in a direction we are not used to going. Too many of us fail to intentionally place Scripture in our thoughts, instead choosing to adopt worldly reasoning.

Psychiatrist Paul Meier, founder of Meier Clinics, often suggests patients (non-Christians too) memorize Scripture. He, too, knows the prescriptive power of the Word of God.[70] Our mind is able to memorize and synthesize life-changing passages of Scripture, enabling us to discern between truth and lies.

Reflect: Read Psalm 7. God's Word is true, whether we feel it or not. He has kept all of his promises and has never failed. Pick any two verses from the Bible and memorize them this week.

We Are Our Memories

If we're going to talk about our mind, we must talk about our memories. When I became a Christian, God pushed the delete key marked "sins," but there wasn't a delete key for my memory bank. Everything, all spiritual, emotional, and physical information stored in my mind before Jesus Christ is still in there, written on my hard drive.

Scientists have found toxic thoughts build toxic memories. Once a thought is received, a memory is built. If the memory is healthy, you benefit. If the memory is bad, you hurt every time you access it.

For example, if a child doesn't have consistent or love-based care, she fails to build up a database of good memories and positive feelings of being loved. That data creates a hole in her soul, which she carries into adulthood. Instead of being comforted by pleasant memories of meaningful relationships, she feels battered and hopeless.

Memories make up our personality—in effect how we react to circumstances, to people, to pain and to joy. We often repress what we don't want to think about, but that memory is still there. God knows when and how to retrieve the memories. We can't change a memory, but we can change how we think about that memory. We will be hostages of our past unless we choose to learn to manage them. We come before him and submit the bad memories so he may heal us. We ask him to bring the bad memories to the surface in order to mend the toxicity as only he can.

You can direct and control your memories by choosing which memories to focus on. Beautiful memories help us feel secure and happy. This is a practice of guarding our heart. Here are some ways you might do this.

If you are experiencing difficulty in the relationship with your mother or your husband or your child, go back into time and recollect the memory of happier times. Why did you first love them in the first place? Reattach yourself to that love. This will begin to enhance the bond between you.

If it's a parent, regardless of how they hurt or failed you, they gave you life instead of aborting you. Be thankful for that. Most likely they had their own struggles and pain, some of which you may never understand because they lived in a different time.

When we fail to guard our hearts and mind or when a trying circumstance rears its devilish head, we may find ourselves drifting from God. It is in that moment of spiritual attack we need to pull up a spiritual memory. Begin to collect spiritual memories.

Reflect: Write down the answers to these questions describing them in detail.

1. Recollect a time that joy permeated your life when you first became a Christian.

2. What commitments have you made to God to show him your love?

3. What vows has God made to you? [This requires Bible study]

4. Recall the exhilaration of experiencing a time when you came to understand a new dimension of God's nature.

5. Begin to write down, date, and collect all answers to prayer—no matter how small.

6. Think of incidences where God has been at work in your relationships—when you felt most competent, happy, and connected to others.

R.E.S.I.S.T. Recap

Recognize the power and intended results of Satan's thought dart attacks. Work to protect your brain, making it less vulnerable to outside spiritual attacks.

Embrace brain-care and mental imagery giving you the power to change a toxic thought to an affirmative and harmless thought.

Submit any bad memories to Jesus. Make a promise to God, and your family if necessary, that you will begin to work to change how you think about a particular toxic memory that is an obstacle today. Name that memory, bringing it into submission!

Identify & Interrogate who you are today. Interrogate your memory bank, seeking to replace negative memories with new positive spiritual memories. Put a plan into place to keep a record of all encouraging and hopeful memories.

Set your mind and heart on God by intentionally placing Scripture in your mind to repel Satan's fiery arrows. What plan have you devised for daily Scripture reading?

Thank and Praise God for the times he has been at work in your relationships—when you have felt most competent, happy, and connected to others. Praise him for his creation—your incredible mind and brain!

What's On Your Mind?

People ask me how I can stand before the world and talk about my immoral past. My response comes out of Scripture, "My old life, that other person, is dead and gone. My new life, which is my *real* life—even though invisible to spectators—is with Christ in God. *He* is now my life. Anyone united with Jesus Christ gets a fresh start and is created new" (Col. 3:3; 5:17, Msg).

However, this incredible metamorphosis did not happen over night. At first, I believed this miraculous change came at my hand. *I finally got my life together. These self-help books finally worked. I'm fixed!* Satan made sure the glory due God got shoved away under the carpet with all of my dirty secrets. I was free from seventeen years of bulimia but the party girl mindset and lifestyle still held my soul hostage. I unknowingly remained deceived.

Deep inside, I desired to be completely free from these toxic behaviors but still did not do what I wished because I wasn't nourishing myself with God's Word. I didn't put God into my schedule. I still had remnants of my old obsessive-compulsive nature which Satan continued to target.

I wasn't any closer to freedom because I didn't give God access to the old destructive mindholds of the past that needed to be broken down. Years later, for the first time, I completely submitted my will to God—not a part here and a part there, like I had in the past, but all of it.

So often, we try to out-plan God, believing we know what is best for ourselves. All we have is a limited view. God has an unlimited view. He sees every minute detail and knows exactly how to give us the very best of him. Scripture says, "In his heart a man plans his course, but the LORD determines his steps" (Prov. 16:9). The key is letting go of control and allowing God to direct our steps so we may end up right where he wants us—in the middle of his amazing plan for us.

As we walk and build a personal relationship with Jesus, the Holy Spirit begins to show us our unholy habits and thoughts. I was not going to mature until I asked God to reveal why I did what I did. We each have to come face to face with our depraved state before we can take responsibility for our actions.

Over time, the Spirit opened the dungeon door to my past, and I saw all the damage I caused. I tended to blame others for my inept behavior and poor choices. Jesus doesn't accept that answer. Instead he says, "Get up! You are no longer bound in your pain-filled past. You've been set free!" He reminded me that:

> He [God] reached down from on high and took hold of me; he drew me out of deep waters. He rescued me from my powerful enemy [*addiction, obsessive-compulsiveness, self-loathing*], from my foes, who were too strong for me. They confronted me [*the enemy doesn't give up easily*] in the day of my disaster, but the LORD was my support. *He rescued me because he delighted in me.*
>
> Psalm 18:16–19, *my emphasis*

Together we started on an incredible adventure (R.E.S.I.S.T) to clean up the accumulated emotional damage that led to my depression and destructive behaviors. Charles Spurgeon said, "Be not content till the whole mind is deeply and vitally changed in reference to sin."[71] The new mindset began to replace the old. Because I am in Christ, I have authority over my flesh, the world, and Satan! I want to finish my race well—the race God has given me to run.

When we turn our life over to Christ, we face a new dilemma to fulfill the destiny God intended for our life. We must learn to see ourselves the way God sees us. It that easy? No! It means we must work to overcome the emotional and physical scars we received while the devil had possession of our soul. We must learn to basically reprogram our thinking with God's thinking.

I embraced what God had to show me, which broke the bond of denial. He had a different definition of purging, which leads to freedom. Eventually, after purging out the hurts and sin and settling my inner disputes, the Cover Girl mask broke into irreparable pieces taking away the need for living a life of lies.

No longer under the devil's thumb, I finally understood in my heart and believed that apart from God I could do nothing. I saw myself as his valued child. He didn't see me as that soiled and damaged woman. He saw me as one of his beautiful children, whom he loved greatly. I had been broken and bruised by the sins of this world, but now lay in his arms joyfully sobbing "Abba Father!" (*Abba* is an intimate word that denotes the close relationship between a child of God and himself.)

If God could reach down and help me climb out of my pit and change my mindset, he can certainly do the same for you wherever you are. A mere mustard seed of faith can transform a toxic situation into an opportunity for God's amazing grace.

It is easy to praise God for his healing touch, his blessings, and grace. How often do you praise God for the tough times? David proclaimed, "Praise be to the Lord, for he has heard my cry for mercy. The Lord is my strength and my shield; my heart trusted in Him, and I am helped; therefore my heart greatly rejoices, and with my song I will praise him" (Ps. 28: 6–7). David also said he would praise the Lord in the morning and again at night, which means he was praising him all the time (Ps. 92:2).

If we are to praise God from morning to night, that means we are to praise him when we are in a dark and troubled place. David praised the Lord because he was his strength and shield— his protection in times of trouble. The true test of faith in God is the ability to praise him for being our protector and provider when things are hard.

Reflect: Praise God for two things he has recently done for you. Praise him for the present and the future. Look up the following five Scriptures in the Psalms and read each one out loud: Psalm 26:12; 69:30; 75:1; 92:1–2; and 105:1.

How You Feel Matters

Women of Faith speaker, Marilyn Meberg, says "emotions don't have brains." She'll also tell you as a former therapist that we can't afford to ignore our emotions.[72] Emotion is God-given and the spice that gives life flavor. Our emotions drive our wills. Often we will be required to put our emotions aside in order to do what is right in God's eyes. But let's not forget, emotion is evidence of life. Jesus had emotions.

Emotions themselves are neither amoral. It is what we do with them and how we respond to them that can be judged as good or bad, righteous or evil. Most of our feelings about ourselves are built into us in childhood.

If we were fortunate to have loving parents who conveyed our worth, and if we grew up in a safe environment with positive relationships with peers, teachers, and role models, then it is likely we will feel reasonably good about ourselves. The child becomes endowed with emotional intelligence that serves rather than enslaves that child for the rest of their life.[73]

However, if we grew up faced with negative influences, such as ongoing rejection or teasing or issues of abandonment, we're most likely to have low self-esteem. If toxic emotional memories pile up in early childhood, physiologically, brain chemicals hijack the rest of the brain by flooding it with strong and inappropriate emotions.

Spiritually, Satan sends out his army when we are children and unbelievers. Using influences such as our family, friends, teachers, or other professionals, his motive is to shoot lies into our little minds as early and as often as possible. This is when we're sensitive and gullible. Unknowingly, a parent is often the culprit. How kids perceive and then respond to words and action is different than adults. After swimming into a wall (ouch!), Amy believed Mom when she laughed and said, "You'll never be good at anything."

Unfortunately, shame often emerges as a feeling, usually taught by family members. We usually don't clarify what we are saying to them. We actually impact their brain chemistry in an adverse way. Children are too immature to understand the battle going on in their minds, so they believe the lies.

I assume my child knows I love her when I tell her she looks hideous wearing pink-striped pants with a flowered orange and green sweater or when I tell my son not to count on ever being a star athlete. My dad *playfully* teased me when I got my first bra and again when I started my period. I was devastatingly embarrassed.

Teenage girls are furious with parents who don't respond with the perfect answer! And dads, being male, don't usually get this. These types of comments can impact a child's self-image and become mindholds.

It is important we learn to experience our emotions openly and honesty. It is difficult to have interpersonal relationships if we don't. "Emotions are like messengers from the front lines of the battle zone. Our tendency is to kill the messenger. But if we listen carefully, we will learn how to fight the war successfully" (Dr. Dan Allender).[74]

Some people are able to express their emotions freely. Some aren't. Perhaps they have been taught that showing emotion is a sign of weakness or being whiney. Don't discount your feelings. Jesus, himself, experienced strong emotions, and he gives us the God-confidence to do the same.

Reflect on this: The Bible tells us God "set his seal of ownership on us, and put his Spirit in our hearts…" (2 Cor. 1:22). "You were marked in him with a seal, the promised Holy Spirit" (Eph. 1:13). This means you belong to God. Marked with a seal suggests possession and security. Jesus said, "I give them eternal life, and they shall never perish; no one can snatch them out of my hand" (John 10:28).

This means Satan's fiery dart may take a hold of your mind or body, but he cannot penetrate your spirit because it is sealed! You may mess up, but you belong to the Father forever! You are a very significant person! Understanding and owning your identity in

Christ is absolutely essential to your success at living the victorious life as a Christian

It's Alive!

One day I was navigating through a women's Bible study when my abortion experience surfaced. I felt intense pressure to make a choice. I could keep this traumatic experience buried, or I could step out in faith and embrace what Jesus wanted to show me. At first I declined. *That happened so long ago. It has no effect on me now. It's no big deal. I've been forgiven.* God knew I was fighting to deny the pain.

Repressing toxic feelings is how we temporarily deal with our problems. However, they do not go away. As we have learned, painful memories are toxic to the soul. They are stored up in multiple centers in the brain. If those memories are about past events, they remain alive in the present and effect what we do and who we are. We usually say, "I see no reason for bringing up the past. Why beat a dead horse?"

Why? Because we can bury the memories, but we're burying something alive. That's kind of gruesome! What we may not realize is certain events in the past may still influence our present. We examine those events so we can determine the extent to which they are alive. Refusal to do so keeps one trapped.

Through self-examination of the unconscious, we become aware of beliefs shaped by our past. Digging them up, with the help of God and perhaps a professional, frees us to develop new thoughts and beliefs. If we don't develop new thoughts and beliefs, our only choice is to follow the old ways, the old self.

God will, in his time, allow us to retrieve the buried memories and heal them with the truth. I eventually chose to reopen this old wound. With God's guidance, I opened the casket. The only way God could begin the healing process was to completely break me down. When we feel that sense of brokenness and humility, then we are ready to receive the power of God's grace that comes alive, transforming our lives.

Suppression and denial destabilizes our brain's chemistry and expels toxic waste! When stress prevents molecules of emotions from flowing freely, our autonomic processes (digestion, breathing, immunity, blood flow) collapses. This causes the suppressed toxic emotion to become an emotional mindhold, disrupting our relationship with God and others.

Reflect: What might God want to begin to open up in your life?

~~~

R.E.S.I.S.T. Recap

Recognize that change and maturity only happen as you build a personal relationship with Jesus. Ask the Holy Spirit to show you your unholy habits and thoughts. Learn to recognize exactly how you give Satan access to your thoughts.

Embrace all toxic thinking, breaking any bond of denial or shame or guilt. You may mess up, but never forget you still belong to the Father. Own your identity in Christ. It is absolutely essential to your success at living the victorious life as a Christian.

Submit each negative situation or thought to Jesus, and in his name, tell Satan, "I'm Jesus's daughter. You have no power over me. Be gone!" Your goal is to automatically think Scripture when faced with a TAD or other type of attack.

Identify & Interrogate—Courage asks God to *reveal the whys.* Identify your masked facades. Is this particular mask permanent or do you only put it on in certain situations? God can work with your honest pain.

Set your mind and heart on God, which will make it easier to take your thoughts captive and then give them to him. Put the suggested steps into place so you will be better able to examine each thought against the standard of thinking God has set for you.

Thank and Praise God that he will never reject or hurt you! Also, praise God for the tough times, which he is using to mold you more and more into his unique vessel.

Toxic Temptation

Pastor Jim was livid when he found a receipt for a $250 dress. He yelled at his wife, "How could you do this!"

She replied, "I don't know. I was standing in the store looking at the dress on sale. Then I found myself trying it on. It was like the devil was whispering to me, *You look great in that dress. Buy it! You can make the monthly payments.*

"You know how to deal with Satan. Like Jesus, tell him, 'Get behind me, Satan!' (Matt. 16:23)" Frustrated, she said, "I did. But then he said, 'It looks great from back here. Buy it!' So I did!"

People have been battling temptation since the fall. Playwright Oscar Wilde said, "I can resist anything except temptation."[75] Actress Mae West said, "I generally avoid temptation unless I can't resist it."[76] Temptation is usually anything labeled "off-limits." The term is used in a loose sense to describe actions that indicate a lack of self-control or something that allures, excites, and seduces a person. Personally, I am often tempted to be envious or competitive of other successful women.

Temptation is the classic way Satan operates by enticing believers into sin, which is why he is called "the tempter" (1 Thess. 3:5). When temptation enters our hearts and minds, we either deal with it, gaining mastery over it, or allow it to lead to sinful actions. Temptations come at unexpected moments. Satan watches for distraction, fatigue, anger, hunger, weakness, or loneliness, and then attacks with a tempting offer. It is at that point we make a choice: to let him in or shut him out. The time between the initial temptation and our chosen response is critical. St. Ambrose said, "The devil's snare does not catch you, unless you are first caught by the devil's bait."[77]

Every Christian is tempted, including the saints of the Bible.

Temptation is part of every human being's experience. Who would have thought we'd uncover murder in Moses, drunkenness in Noah, adultery *and* murder in David, and cursing in Job? If God leaves us to ourselves, suddenly and scandalously sin breaks out, even in the holiest men.

The *existence* of a tempting or sinful thought is quite different than the *action* of that thought. To succumb to the temptation is to surrender one's heart and mind to the devil, giving him a foothold. The moment we are tempted to get our physical or emotional need met in a way that is not conforming to Christ, we are at the threshold of a major decision. For example: The cashier gives you fifty dollars change instead of five dollars. What do you think?

1. It's a gift from God, so I will keep it.
2. It's a gift from God, so I will share it.
3. I will alert the cashier to the error.

The Lord said to Cain, "If you do not do what is right, sin is crouching at your door; it desires to have you, but you must master it" (Gen. 4:7). At that precise moment of conviction, we must choose to master the sin crouching at the doorway of our minds.

Today, temptation's lure is money, food, power, and sensuality. The flesh is never satisfied. It always wants more ... and now! I once worked for a start-up software company. The president carefully handpicked a small team that could lead his company into Fortune 500. The team worked relentlessly, traveling all over the world, developing and selling their software. They worked together well and knew one another intimately, spending more time with one another than their own families. One day the president told the team that one of them would leave the company for the lure of money, stock options, and prestige that comes with a key position at a larger software company. Offended, each person vowed, "Not I! I'd never betray this company!"

This was exactly what each disciple said to Jesus when he confronted them: "I tell you the truth, one of you will betray me" (Mark 14:17–18). Each thought, *Never! I'm loyal to my Lord!* Yet, Jesus looked at them and said, "It is one of the Twelve" (Mark 14:20). During the culmination to Jesus's death, the disciples did things they never thought they'd do. But Jesus knew. James said that temptation is the pull of man's own evil thoughts and wishes, which lead to evil actions (James 1:14–15)—man's flesh.

In the pressure of the moment, the mind and heart does surprising things, which is why we are counseled to guard them. We have not sinned until we make the choice to entertain the tempting thought and then follow through. But with every temptation, God also provides an escape so we won't have to yield to it (1 Cor. 10:13).

God has revealed his will in Scripture so we should not be confused about doing the right thing. Have you picked up the theme here? Your power to confront and conquer is found in God's Word, the Holy Bible.

Reflect: Is Jesus warning you of an area in your life which you might easily fall? What one new thing can you do to protect your mind from this temptation?

The Temptation of Jesus

In her journal (October 1866) Hannah Whitall Smith wrote, "The Lord has been teaching me in many ways lately about my utter weakness in the presence of temptation."

Troubled, Hannah felt she had no more power over sin than when she was first converted. "My own efforts have been worse than useless." Then the indwelling Christ spoke to her, and she realized Jesus, too, resisted temptation. He did it through the power of the Holy Spirit. "I realize that Christ dwells in my heart by faith and that He is able and willing to subdue all things to himself."

Jesus said to his disciples, "Hard trials and temptations are bound to come" (Luke 17:1, Msg.). He understands how we feel under the weight of temptation. He took on all the limitations of human flesh and was tempted in every way we are. He faced the tempter and overcame the adversity. The Apostle Matthew gives an account of Jesus's temptation in Matthew 4:1–11.

After the baptism at the Jordan River, Jesus publicly embraced his Messianic role. Satan quickly unleashed three massive assaults. The Bible says, "Jesus was led by the Spirit into the desert to be tempted by the devil. After fasting forty days and forty nights, he was hungry." God had just introduced Jesus as his Son, whom he loved and was very pleased with (Matt. 3:17). Why would the Holy Spirit toss Jesus out into the wilderness to face temptation? I also wonder how Satan appeared to Jesus? Scripture doesn't say.

This sounds like a repeat of what happened to Eve and Adam. Jesus submitted to the leading of the Spirit in order to take on temptation. When God is leading us, it is a test (James 1:13). When Satan is leading us, it is temptation, even though following God's lead may take us into places where we'll be tempted or attacked (Ps. 23:4). God's testing is intended to strengthen our character, whereas Stan's temptations are designed to destroy our character and relationships.

"When the forty days ended, Jesus grew very faint and hungry for he had eaten nothing." Satan remembered how he had tempted Eve and caused her to listen to his words. Adam and Eve were deceived. Perhaps the Messiah (the second Adam) could be.

The situation was primed for food to be a powerful temptation tool. Satan intended to thwart Jesus' dependence on his Father by causing him to use his own resources to meet his need for food. *Your own Father has allowed you to go hungry! If you have a desire, it deserves to be fulfilled!*

Satan said, "If you really are the Son of God, command that these stones become loaves of bread." He assumed Jesus would surely yield to this temptation and tried to disprove he was God's Son. Satan's fiery darts of doubt were aimed directly at God.

Jesus answered, "It is written: Man shall not live by bread only, but by every word of God." Jesus attacked back by quoting Scripture (Deut. 8:3). He could have turned the stones to bread. Although he was hungry and faint, Jesus would not use his great power to please himself. Satan soon saw he could not cause Jesus to yield to such a temptation, so he tried another tactic.

Jesus did not use his divine power to counterattack Satan. He used the same weapon that is available to us—the Word of God. Scripture is the only reliable guide we have to function properly as a human in a broken world. It is penetrating, scrutinizing our desires; therefore, we should test our thinking against what Scripture says is truth.

Reflect: As a believer, we have the power of the Holy Spirit within us to teach us the truths of God's Word (John 16:13–15). How are you making and taking the time to read and study the Bible? Do you find you need help? Do not fear asking for help.

The Second Temptation

Satan hoped to tempt Jesus into testing God's Word with the second temptation. Taking Jesus to the uppermost part of the temple in Jerusalem, he said, "If you expect people to believe that you are really God's Son you must show some great sign. Now cast yourself down to the ground, and trust God to protect you and keep your bones from being broken; for in the Scripture he has promised that angels will bear you up and not allow any harm to befall you."

Satan uses Scripture to tempt Jesus, quoting the Bible accurately (Ps. 91:11,12). Satan knows the Bible far better than we do. How do we resist? As Jesus did, "It is also written ..." We quote Scripture back.

Cherie was told all of her life that she'd never amount to anything. She claimed everything she touched fell apart. One day she was reading in Romans, "Does not the potter have the right to make out of the same lump of clay some pottery for noble purposes and some for common use?" (Rom. 9:21)

Cherie interpreted the verse to mean that God intentionally creates some people to be blessed and successful and others to be cursed and failures. She believed she was the latter. Scripture confirmed what her family had told her all her life. She believed a lie that came right out of the Bible. She knew the potter was God, but what she didn't know was that Paul was addressing a group of Christians who mixed pride, bigotry, and fleshly works with Christ's Word. Paul's desire was to wean his readers away from self-sufficiency.

Paul was telling the Romans that God, the Creator, has full rights over his creation (Rom. 9:20). We humans have no basis to question the acts of God. Scripture clearly tells us we lack the capacity to grasp God's infinite mind or the way he intervenes in our lives. He is not accountable to us. In Romans 9:22–24, the point is that God's judgments and decision are ultimately a display of God's grace and mercy.

This interpretation is ninety degrees apart from Cherie's understanding. Satan always masquerades his lies as God's truth. He enjoys taking verses out of context to prove his false beliefs. This is why it is so important to have a proper grasp of Scripture if we are to detect and defeat him.

Scripture is a brutally honest about life—the good, the bad, the ugly. It can also be taken out of context very easily. It is important that when we start our study of the Scriptures, in addition to our own individual devotional time, we are learning from reputable pastors and teachers. King Solomon wisely advised: "For lack of guidance a nation falls, but *many advisers* make victory sure" (Prov. 11:14, *my emphasis*).

Reflect: We must memorize God's Word. Jesus didn't have a concordance with him. He reached into his memory bank and selected Deuteronomy, quoting three verses to silence Satan. Memorization isn't just for children. It is for every believer. It's our sword of the Spirit (Eph. 6:17). If we don't have God's Word in our memory, then the Holy Spirit is unable to bring it to our minds when we are under attack.

The Third Temptation

Satan desires worship, and the third temptation of Jesus was in regard to power and wealth. Today, he tempts us with power and success, appealing to human pride. Entrepreneur and millionaire Donald Trump received a great deal of publicity following the success of his reality television show, *The Apprentice*. Ambition and drive are not bad qualities, as long as our motives are pure and we are not driven to obtain a perishable crown (1 Cor. 9:25).

Satan took Jesus to the top of a high mountain and caused him to see all the kingdoms of the world. "I can give them to any one I choose. Now I will give them to you if only you will fall down and worship me." *You can be a super power through me!* Satan is actually the ruler of this domain. Today these kingdoms lie within his power. But one day he will lose full control.

Jesus lambasted him, "Get away from me, you evil one! For it is written in the Scriptures that the Lord God is the only Being who should be worshiped." We can deride Satan too. Shout, "Get out of here! Leave me alone Satan!" Our power is the same Jesus relied on, the power coming from God's Word and the Holy Spirit, which is our authority to tell Satan to get lost.

Then Satan left Jesus alone. He could find no way to crowd sin into the pure heart of the Son of God. The angels came from heaven and supplied Jesus' needs. His basic needs were taken care of—not through Satan's devices, but through the kingdom's. Jesus faced what you face—physical, emotional, and spiritual temptation by Satan.

Heaven must have rejoiced at Jesus's victory over the evil one! In the book of Luke this story concludes, "When the devil had finished all this tempting, he left him until an opportune time" (Luke 4:13).

Jesus, filled with the power of the Spirit, stood up to Satan's temptation and defeated him. Then he began his public ministry. But Satan would be back. Ever vigilant, he strikes again. That is why Jesus taught us to pray, "Lead us not into temptation, but deliver us from the evil one" (Matt. 6:13).

Reflect: What similarities do you see in regard to the temptations of Adam and Eve and Jesus's three temptations? What about your temptations? Pray that God keeps you safe from yourself—your flesh and ego, the temptations of the world, and the devil.

Sensuous Samson and Deceptive Delilah

Picture a tabloid heading: "Samson Loves Delilah, But Does She Love Him?"

In the Bible, Samson is a Herculean figure who leads Israel for twenty years. Today he'd be a superstar athlete or an action movie star, and probably on the cover of *Sports Illustrated.* He was granted tremendous strength through the spirit of the Lord to combat his enemies and perform heroic feats unachievable by ordinary men. Delilah is described as one of several dangerous temptresses in the Old Testament (Judg. 13–16).

Succumbing to temptation, Samson divulged the secret of his strength to the temptress Delilah. The Bible reads, "Having put him to sleep on her lap, she called a man to shave off the seven braids of his hair, and so began to subdue him. And his strength left him … Then the Philistines seized him, gouged out his eyes and took him down to Gaza. Binding him with bronze shackles, they set him to grinding in the prison" (Judg. 16:19, 21). *Ouch!*

Samson ended up becoming a slave (literally) to his own sin. One of the signs of a heart that has shifted from God is the absence of spiritual power. If you are like Samson, you will not be immediately aware that God's power has left you. Only after he tried to defeat his enemies did Samson recognize something was wrong. He prevailed over the Philistines in every battle, except this last one.

When we yield to temptation, we hurt ourselves, other people, and we grieve God. Every relationship is affected. Businessman Warren Buffett said, "It takes twenty years to build a reputation and five minutes to ruin it. If you think about that, you'll do things differently."[78]

As we grow in Christ we can count on facing opposition. Recognize temptation as being necessary and vital for your maturity. It is always packaged in the form of choice: who shall I worship? The Creator or the creation; God or some god I design; Jesus or myself? As we seek to follow God, temptations will inevitably increase. Every temptation is an opportunity for us to grow closer to God.

Our first response to a known temptation is to guard our mind. "Our defeat or victory begins with what we think, and if we guard our thoughts we shall not have much trouble anywhere else along the line" (Vance Havner).[79]

We must work to protect and watch over what we allow into our mind. We must desire to keep out of sin's way and detach ourselves from temptation. We examine our thinking, attitude, behavior, and then weigh those choices against potential consequences, setting our eyes on Jesus, not on the temptation.

Second, we submit any tempting thought or impulse to the obedience of Christ. Temptation can be so powerful we cannot resist without the help of the Holy Spirit. He is the only one who can give us the power to take that temptation into obedience. There will be times when we miss, even ignore, the prompting of the Spirit warning us that God is not pleased with the direction our thoughts and feelings are going.

When we finally see the err of our ways, we repent. "Change your mind and attitude to God and turn to him so he can cleanse away your sins and send you wonderful times of refreshment from the presence of the Lord" (Acts 3:19, TLB).

Third, if we continue to fall into the same trap, we ask God why—we interrogate. Moses told his people, "Consider the generations long past. Ask your father and he will tell you, your elders, and they will explain to you" (Deut. 32:7).

We must understand our roots. Termed *generational sin,*

Scripture asserts that God will visit the sins of the parents upon the children (Ex. 20:5). Some of us inherited our troubles. Alcoholism frequently recurs in one's children. It may be racist mindset. Most child abusers were abused themselves. Whatever the reason, thank God he will forgive you over and over again. And he will give you the power to break "the curse" so you do not pass it on to your children.

Reflect: Read and meditate on 1 Corinthians 10:13. Pray: "Lord, today I will make a thousand small, consequential, and trivial choices. Help me to choose the one thing needed for a richer, more vital life in you. Amen."

Temptation and Imagination

Charles Spurgeon confessed he wrestled with his imagination, "Those who have a fair share of imagination know what a difficult thing it is to control. You cannot restrain it. My imagination has taken me down to the vilest kennels and sewers of earth."[80]

Neurophysiologists have discovered that the brain responds to mental images as if the activity were actually happening. There is no difference in the brain wave whether an athlete is swinging a bat or only seeing an image of himself doing so.[81]

Neuroeconomists found that imagining a future purchase is almost as good as getting it. Your brain gets a zing whether you purchase or imagine it.[82] So the next time you are tempted to buy those cute black shoes, instead, imagine yourself wearing them. You'll get a zing and save yourself some money.

The same goes for the not-so desirable thoughts. Now we understand why Jesus equated sinful thoughts with sinful action.

Paul taught in 2 Corinthians 10:3–5 (ASV):

> For though we walk in the flesh, we do not war according to the flesh (for the weapons of our warfare are not of the flesh, but mighty before God to the casting down of strongholds), casting down imaginations, and every

high thing that is exalted against the knowledge of God, and bringing every thought into captivity to the obedience of Christ.

Paul mentions three things: strongholds, imaginations, and a thought. A thought unchecked becomes our imagination, which is the action or process of forming images or concepts. Those images become our self-talk.

When an image or thought says *failure, loser, fat,* that becomes the picture you see of yourself—your image. An image can become a mindhold. My image was that I had to be beautiful and youthful in order to be accepted and considered a success. My mindhold was insecurity in my appearance and who I really was.

Most toxic thought patterns arise from three common, yet incorrect, beliefs:

1. I must do well (we each have our own definition of success).

2. You must treat me humanely and with kindness.

3. The world must be easy.

These are toxic because in this world no one does well all the time, everyone is mistreated at some time, and life is not easy or fair. On the surface, a thought like "I must do well" seems positive, but only when you look at it closely and analyze the feelings it generates can you see how it is as an accusation in disguise.

Demanding unrealistic performance from ourselves, and others, puts our minds and bodies in stress mode, affecting our health. We have a choice at this point: take the thought captive and toss it out or let the thought through, wreaking havoc on our minds and bodies.

Personally, I am continually tempted with diet and anti-aging products. Satan often whispers, *If you were thinner and younger looking, you'd have more opportunities!* If we repeatedly fall to the same temptation, our response is interrogation. *Why,*

Lord, is my weight and my appearance still so significant to me? You've already blessed me with enormous opportunities.

The answer: I've been brainwashed by this culture! Advertisements promise: *Lose weight no matter how much you eat and without diet or exercise! Try our truly remarkable anti-ageing cream, which has been described as the fountain of youth.* I must identify and take captive these types of false messages and replace them with truth.

Truth: most diet and anti-aging product promises are misleading and downright counterfeit. Approximately 95 percent of all people who diet gain their weight back and most women don't see their wrinkles disappear. I can personally attest to that! The truth is found in 2 Corinthians 4:16 and 1 Peter 3:3–4. Beauty in God's eyes comes from your inner self, which is being renewed daily.

Reflect: With the Holy Spirit's help, I began identifying the stinking thinking, and then I tossed it out, over and over again. This is what it means to take captive every thought, including all false beliefs and messages, to Jesus. We put that negative thought where it belongs—behind bars. We get rid of it. Toss it out!

Capturing A Toxic Thought

Science's verdict is in: there is a connection between taking our thoughts captive and giving them to Jesus with the healing of our body and our lives.

In Paul's day there were many false apostles spreading deceptive truths, as there are today. He was requesting the church's complete obedience. Obedience is usually an act of behavior. Every behavior begins with a thought, so by bringing our thought captive into obedience, the right actions follow.

After being captured, every thought must be sifted through the filter system in our brain. Your brain allows you to select approximately 15–35 percent of what you read, hear, and see while getting rid of the remaining 65–85 percent.[83] It's got a large trash or recycle bin. If we build our mind with Scripture and godly thinking, then everything that goes through that sifter that is not scriptural, or truth, will set off our mental alarm. We reject it and toss it into the trash bin.

Physiologically, toxic thoughts upset the chemical balance in your brain, putting your body in a harmful state. Your brain actually will weigh down your whole body, mind, and spirit. Your brain grows heavy and optimal functioning is disrupted.[84] The only way to prevent this from happening is by sifting through the toxic information and tossing it out. When you set your mind on Jesus and consciously take control of your thought life, it doesn't take long for the positive benefits to kick in.

For a long time I struggled with public prayer. One day I asked God to reveal the *why*. I realized public prayer made me uncomfortable because I compared myself to those who pray so well. I was convinced in my mind that as I prayed I would be graded by those listening, and what an enormous task! This had Satan's fingerprints all over it.

God showed me that every time I followed my imagination I was separating myself from him. Prayer on behalf of others is a privilege! And if you feel this way, let me assure you—no one is comparing or grading you. If they are, they are grading the Holy Spirit, the one who is guiding you!

This goes back to faith versus fear. When I relied on my own reasoning and emotions, I feared praying publicly. When I captured these thoughts and tossed them out, I decided, by faith, I would pray publicly. It would be a positive, rewarding experience.

Research shows that an environment enriched with positive thinking leads to changes in the brain's cortex in a relatively short amount of time. Research has also discovered one of the benefits of controlling your thoughts is you become more intelligent![85] I try to stretch myself by taking risks and reading more.

Reflect: What two new things can you do to stretch your mind positively?

R.E.S.I.S.T. Recap

Recognize temptation is lurking behind every bush, demons are opposing your every step, and your flesh is continually making treasonous advances trying to undercut your spiritual progress. Your response: guard your mind with a Bible reading plan.

Embrace the Word of God to fight temptation. Be aware Satan knows the Bible far better than you do. He enjoys taking verses out of context to prove his false beliefs. Carve out time each day to learn and rest in God's Word.

Submit all tempting thoughts and impulses to the obedience of Christ. Actively acknowledge each toxic thought (take it captive) and then proactively submit it to Christ. Those thoughts no longer define you. They've been tossed out.

Identify & Interrogate—Get into the habit of examining your thinking and behavior. What incorrect beliefs have you identified so far? With the Holy Spirit's help, prayerfully identify any painful or stinking thinking. Learn to sift through the toxic information and toss each toxic thought out—over and over again.

Set your mind and heart on God so that when Satan strikes you can pull up memorized Scripture. God's Word is your sword. Make a commitment to work to consciously take control of your thought life.

Thank and Praise God that the extent of each temptation is controlled by him. "Our temptations can be turned into stepping stones leading to nobility of character" (Herbert Lockyer).[86]

Acidic Accusation

Pew Research finds 81 percent of young adults say getting rich is their most important life goal; 51 percent say the same about being famous.[87] Each year, over one-hundred thousand young guys and girls audition for *American Idol,* and dream: *If I'm rich and famous, everyone will idolize and accept me. Life will be easy!* Contestants pin their hopes and futures on four fallible judges and an erratic American public.

The desire to attain celebrity seems to be driven by a desire to not be plain and ordinary, which is comical because God created mostly ordinary-looking people! The desire for fame and riches lurks in the human heart, but in reality, that desire is really seeking a deeper hunger only God can satisfy.

The truth about accusation is that Satan is at work behind the scene creating these feelings. He likes to remind us of our unworthiness, failures, and sin, even though God sees us as completely acceptable. Ask yourself, "What beliefs actively shape the way I live? What assumptions do I make? What expectations do I carry within my heart? These are areas that may need to be submitted to God.

Many of us wouldn't say we're seeking superstar status, but find ourselves basing our self-worth on how others see us and our accomplishments. Some call it "the rejection syndrome." Our culture sets us up for hurt and rejection, which is why so many of us become driven to win and be perfect. We become perfectionists and performers, living a life we cannot sustain.

The biography on the back cover of my first book began: "Author Kimberly Davidson is a woman who wears many hats. She is…" My hats were listed. The intended reaction: *Pretty impressive!* The real reaction should be: *Fool!*

Like generations of women who have gone before me, I too

made the same mistake of taking on what God did not gift or intend for me to take on. When the church I attended found out I was a seminary student, they said, "Boy, do we have a job for you! We want you to direct women's ministries."

Instead of standing up for myself and telling the board that leading this ministry was not what I believed God called me to do *and* taking this to God in prayer to seek his will, my need to please people and perform kicked in. So I accepted. To back out would have been far worse. I thought, *Perhaps this is God's will?* For three years I was frustrated and bitter. I felt very guilty for feeling that way. At one point my leg broke out with shingles. *If I don't put on a happy face, Jesus will be disappointed in me.* Wrong!

Moses finally told the Israelites, "You are a great burden for me to carry all by myself" (Deut. 1:9, TLB). He knew his limits. Learning to respect boundaries, our own and other people's, can eliminate much of the stress that hinders relationships. Our journey on this earth is not about fixing or controlling others, but loving them and treating them as we want to be loved and treated. However, many Christians focus so much on being loving and giving that they forget their own limitations. (I recommend Drs. Henry Cloud and John Townsend's book, *Boundaries.*)

Everybody has their own beliefs about how people should respond to them and why. Some of us feel we were picked on unfairly. Others blame their parent's childrearing style. How we act or react depends on how we perceive our past and the accusations we wear. We also make choices about how we will respond.

There are three major accusatory mindholds that mold our masks: people pleasing, perfectionism and performance, and victimization. Each one affects us personally and affects every relationship. Each mindhold says in a roundabout way, *it is all about me.* Therefore, it must be broken.

Reflect: As you consider each mindhold as it relates to you, interrogate it. Ask God to show you what might be causing it and what may be hindering you from breaking it. We want to submit and then break down any mindhold that blocks our relationship with God and others.

The People Pleaser

Mindhold #1: I must be loved or approved by every significant person in my life. I depend on others for my value. I am a people-pleaser.

Almost all women understand what it means to be a people pleaser. Our longing for acceptance and relationship often leads us to ignore our own needs because our perceptions have become distorted. It's been said for every one positive comment made, a child receives ten negative comments. In school, students hear seven or more negative statements from their teachers for every one positive statement. It takes seven compliments to undo the effects of just one criticism.

No wonder we grow up feeling we need to do whatever it takes to be accepted. We may even feel pressure from our church community to measure ourselves according to a certain image. In the Old Testament Saul obeyed the people instead of God because he feared people more than God (1 Sam.15:24). That was a great insult to God.

If we are living to make sure others like or love us, we give them the power to determine our self-worth. I must constantly remind myself I work for God, not people. To take every thought captive means refusing to allow other people's approval or disapproval of me dominate my thinking. We should not trying to please men but God (1 Thess. 2:4). Luckily, God doesn't care how well I sing or what I look like on the outside, and he doesn't play favorites.

A. W. Tozer said that if the devil comes to you and whispers that you are no good, don't argue with him, instead, remind him: "Regardless of what you say about me, I must tell you how the Lord feels about me. He tells me that I am so valuable to him that he gave himself for me on the cross!"[88] I'm perfect just the way I am!

Reflect: Anyone who created yesterday's pain does not control tomorrow's potential! Determine that you will please God regardless of the opinions of others. Today God is saying to you:

"This is my Son [*daughter*], whom I love; with him [*her*] I am well pleased" (Matt. 17:5). Do not allow the devil to steal God's heart and unconditional love from you.

The Perfectionist and Performer

Mindhold #2: I must be painstakingly competent and perfect in order to consider myself worthwhile. I must work hard to be loved. Therefore, I must be a super-sheep. I am a perfectionist and/or a performer.

We live in a world that defines a person's value and worth by productivity. How much we get done and how well we do it are the benchmarks of a successful day. This doesn't come without a cost. One of the leading causes of depression is having standards so high you cannot live up to them.

Defined as *anxious slavery* or *slow suicide,* perfectionists feel they need to prove their value to avoid the threat of rejection. Guilty! "Perfectionism makes us despise ourselves when we spot imperfection, and then we try harder to be perfect which is really a form of narcissism which feeds on foolish pride, and worse, devalues the cross" (Dr. Larry Crabb).[89]

Have you ever noticed a perfectionist usually marries the opposite? A husband who is so organized that he can predict with a fair degree of accuracy when his next shoestring is going to break, inevitably gets paired with a wife who hasn't the foggiest notion what she's going to prepare for dinner at five p.m.

A wife, with an obsession for cleanliness jumps out of bed at one a.m. because she suddenly remembers she forgot to mop up a blob of spilled orange juice from the kitchen floor, marries a clod who comes in from a hunting trip and tracks mud all over the floor she just cleaned. So goes the struggle between perfection and imperfection.

There is a certain amount of tension in every Christian's mind concerning the biblical call to perfection. In one compartment of the brain there's a tug to live up to all the standards of

Kimberly Davidson

Christ, but then on the other side, our attempts to measure up to those standards are always flawed.

How then do we interpret Matthew 5:48, "be perfect, therefore, as your heavenly Father is perfect." The word "perfect" is the Greek word *teleios,* which means "mature, fully developed." It doesn't refer to flawless or moral perfection, but to the kind of love that is like God's love—mature, complete, holy, full of blessing. To be perfect is to seek and work to love others as wholeheartedly as God loves us and fulfill the purpose for which you were made.

The Old Testament speaks of being "upright" and "righteous." Sounds like perfection to me! The upright and righteous are not perfect. They are persons who confess their sin because they hate it and trust God for forgiveness and help.

As a ministry leader often I find myself falling back into the perfection rut, feeling I have to meet some very high expectations. What has been very freeing to me is to realize that when God called me to ministry he knew what he was getting. A couple months down the road he didn't say, "Bad decision. I shouldn't have called her!" Companies say that. People say that. Not God. That's the freedom of grace. You are already completely acceptable to God as imperfect as you are. Thank you Jesus!

God defines personhood and success very differently than our culture does. The measure of our life is not where we live, how we look, or how well we sew or cook. From his perspective, success is measured by what kind of person we are, even in the midst of life's challenges.

God's grace is greater than our imperfections, than our sin, and far greater than Satan (Rom. 5:20–21). "Christ redeemed [*freed*] us from the curse of the law [*the curse of perfectionism*] by becoming a curse for us" (Gal. 3:13, *my emphasis*). Jesus Christ became (past tense) the curse for us, freeing us from all perfectionistic law traps. *Perfection* means a perfect union with God for which we were created.

Reflect: James 3:2 proclaims we all stumble in many ways. Nobody, apart from God, is perfect. People will always fail, disappoint and hurt us. We will make mistakes, even humiliate ourselves. God gives us an incredible gift when we become his daughter—grace. Today, give yourself grace.

⌖

The Victim

Mindhold #3: My past determines my present behavior, and because something once strongly affected my life, it should continue to do so. I'm chained to my past. I am a victim. I blame others. I cannot help the way I am.

Most likely you have a darn good reason to feel this way. The world will tell you the dominating influence in your life is your past. I always found it easier to blame others for my destructive actions. However, all victimization does is create deep mindholds. In this culture, when things go wrong we support the belief that this was done to us by some larger force, as opposed to me bringing it upon myself. This is a recipe for passivity, hopelessness, and helplessness.

Our culture tends to teach and train victims. Father Ken Deasy, a Roman Catholic priest, titled his book *Get Off the Cross—Someone Else Needs the Wood*. We can become content on our cross. The cartoon character Popeye the Sailorman, always settling, his catchphrase was, "I yam what I yam." We tend to get what we expect. These thoughts are a ticket to the road of self-destrucion.

You may have had something traumatic or embarrassing happen to you. Perhaps you feel shame about certain aspects of your family. Or maybe you have some bad or sinful habits you feel humiliated about. Perhaps you have done some things in your past you are ashamed of. Or, maybe you have mistreated others. Your past is not your identity! Scripture promises that Jesus is "able to do immeasurably *more than all we ask or imagine*, according to his power that is *at work within us ...*" (Eph. 3:20, *my emphasis*).

We may not forget the past, but we don't have to be controlled by it. We must stop looking in the rear-view mirror.

Lot's wife looked back to the life she was leaving behind and she turned into a pillar of salt! (Gen. 19:26) Clinging to the past, she was unwilling to completely turn away.

We are responsible human beings, not victims. Studies in the 1970s and 1980s showed the cause of crime is not, as we have been lead to believe, a bad environment or upbringing.90 If we fault our background, then we are not taking responsibility, and worse, there is no need for a Savior.

When I feel like I've been wronged, I think about Christ. He was oppressed and afflicted, yet he never said a word. He was brought as a lamb to the slaughter; and a sheep before its shearers. Yet, Jesus never cried, *Woe is me! Life is so unfair.* He stood silent before the ones condemning him (Isa. 53:7).

We can't alter or delete the past. Instead we focus on what we are becoming. The Holy Spirit is conforming us to the image of Christ and renewing our mind! Henry Ford (Ford Motor Company) said, "Don't find fault, find a remedy."91 The remedy is Christ himself.

We all have stuff that needs to be exposed. And it is absolutely necessary to growing into Christlikeness. But God's Word also says, "Forget the former things; do not dwell on the past. See, I am doing a new thing!" (Isa. 43:18) We need to forget the past and look forward to what lies ahead (Phil. 3:13). When God frees us in an area of bondage, we're done! Satan is the only one who tells you to look backwards. Get goal oriented for the kingdom and start working on using your gifts. Begin to set some goals for your future. What do you have a passion to do?

Accusation versus Conviction

We must learn to differentiate between Satan's accusation and the Holy Spirit's conviction of sin. The word *conviction* basically means exposing and correcting. It is when a firm belief is questioned or judged. It's an uneasy but good feeling.

When the Spirit convicts us, he uses the Word of God

which is often mediated through another Christian, particularly preachers as they proclaim the Word of God. God uses his Word to bring us back into relationship with himself while showing us where and how we need to change our thinking and behavior.

I am honored God invites me to be in the middle of where he is actively working. Not only have I felt honored, I've felt prideful. Satan whispered, *You are really important!* I agreed and would try to slip this information into my conversations.

I began to recognize, because the Holy Spirit was convicting me, that when I inserted my comments about my work, it appeared as honest conversation to the person listening, but my heart was really bragging. It's no different than a name-dropper who casually mentions her recent conversation with the governor.

I interrogated this imprisoned thought, "Lord, Why do I brag about this?"

Because you want to be admired for the work you are doing.

"Admired as in i-dolatry?"

Yes.

Then God took me back to Genesis 3, and the serpent was looking at me eye to eye. *You want to be like God, don't you? Eat the fruit!* My soul froze, not able to believe what God revealed. I had to search my heart and ask that awful question, "Do I want to be like God...play God?"

There's only one God...and I'm not it!

Every time I bragged about what I was doing in ministry, I took a bite of the fruit. Then God revealed more at a later time. I still harbored a certain amount of insecurity—a temptation to break confidentiality in order to feel more important. I confessed my pride. I prayed for victory over this sin and asked God to give me a heart of humility. Throughout this conviction process I never felt condemned.

Reflect: Meditate on this truth: "God has reconciled you by Christ's physical body through death to present *you holy in his sight, without blemish and free from accusation—if* you continue in your faith" (Col. 1:22–23, *my emphasis*).

Nothing but the Truth, So Help Me, God!

Quite often my house is filled with the smell of burnt food (cooking is not my gift). I open the windows, but the smell lingers. Eventually the fresh country air clears it away. It's the same with our toxic thoughts and feelings. We have to open our windows. We let the clean, refreshing air of God's Word circulate through our mind, heart, and soul, replenishing and renewing our whole being. We begin to feel joy again.

The Bible is food, not burnt food, but truth food. It feeds your mind, heart, body, and soul. As you ingest and digest God's Word, it dispels lies, becomes energy for life, like an umbilical cord. It contains the right mixture of nutrients to keep us spiritually alive, nourishing our heart, mind, and body continually.

Like children, the more you eat, the more you grow. As you take it in, it turns into fuel, feeding your brain and thoughts. Our minds are changed by the knowledge God puts into our brains, turning it into fuel which feeds every cell, creating growth.

Unfortunately, the world considers truth optional. God has revealed his desire for all to be saved and to come to the knowledge of the truth (1 Tim. 2:3). God and truth are inseparable. The truth describes how things really are—what's real. It challenges denial and acknowledges fear. Someone once said *truth is like surgery, it may hurt, but it cures.*

What is meant by biblical truth? Both the Father and Jesus are truth (John 7:28; 8:26; 14:6; 17:3)—the opposite of falsehood. From his first contact with Adam and Eve, Satan has been lying to us, persuading us to live in falsehood rather than truth. God sent Jesus into the world to reveal the truth to you and me. Truth is *the* key to mind renewal and it incapacitates our enemy.

Truth can be hard to understand because all human beings are limited in their understanding. This is why we need the Holy Spirit to guide us through the Scriptures into complete truth, away from lies and deception (John 16:13) in order to think, do, and speak what is right.

Jesus said if we follow him we will know the truth [Jesus], and the truth will set us free (John 8:30–32). First we pursue Jesus, coming to know him more intimately, and then we start to follow his will. Truth begins to infuse our minds and hearts ... *then* we are set free. God's Word sets us free as we allow it to nourish our soul.

One afternoon, a pastor spent a couple hours with a dying woman who was very anxious about what was going to happen to her soul. They talked about much of the same things we have talked about. Finally her eyes were opened to the truth and the gospel message. Before she died, she said to the pastor with obvious regrets, "I feel like a louse. I've served Satan all my life and only now at the end have I learned the real truth."

It's never too late. Nothing can quiet the troubled heart and mind like biblical truth—the great doctrines, realities, and assurances of God's Holy Word. As we read his Word each day we ask, "What does God mean by what he says?" It is the task of the interpreter to discern its meaning, and proper interpretation must precede application. "We are not entitled to redefine "truth" to fit our own personal viewpoints, preferences or desires" (John MacArthur).[92]

The Bible does not always equate an encounter with God as a *felt* experience—a spiritual "high." Highs are great when they come, but we truly experience God when we *believe* and have *faith* in what his Word says, and when *hope* is our anchor in his promises. Each time we open our Bible we ask the Holy Spirit to lead and teach us—to help us interpret correctly. He is ready to guide us into all truth (John 15:26; 16:13).

It is one thing to know about truth. It is another to experience the truth being worked throughout your life. Truth produces fruit, but that fruit will have no effect upon your heart unless you accept it and believe with your whole mind. This takes time and depending on your history, might also require professional counseling.

The Bible gives us a clear choice between two roads to travel in life: the way of the flesh, the devil, and the world; or the way of God—of truth and light. The first road may look smoother and like a more direct route, but it is disguised because we run into Satan, who eventually builds mindholds within our soul.

We have to take God's road. It looks bumpier and is more difficult to navigate. It can get pretty steep in some places. And watch out—the devil will even create sinkholes and ice patches. The climb up may even take its toll on our energy level. We may get lonely on this road because there aren't as many people on it. Then we get a glimpse in the rear-view mirror and see there are others following because of our example.

Despite the challenges, God's road is bound for the highest peak. We will make it because God throws us a lifeline from the top. Each day we need to ask God for the strength and ability to R.E.S.I.S.T. the way of the old life and mindset. "You armed me with strength for battle; you made my adversaries bow at my feet" (Ps. 18:39).

Reflect: Not only must we learn and apply truth to our own lives; we must teach and model it to our children and others. Pray for knowledge of truth that will change your life rather than simply filling up your mind. Define truth as it applies to your life today.

R.E.S.I.S.T. Refresher

Recognize Jesus has "given you authority to trample on snakes and scorpions and to overcome all the power of the enemy; nothing will harm you" (Luke 10:19). Notice Jesus didn't say he'd lead you around these evil critters. He gives you the authority and power to stomp them out. But they will be back! When you are exposed to wrong ideas or opportunities or ideologies, trample on them.

Embrace the entire process of self-examination, confession, submission, and repentance. Most of us want to change, are motivated to change, and like the results, but we don't like the process. Embrace change! No longer deny there is a problem or pain.

Submit every conscious thought to Christ. Sift it through your brain in submission to him. Submission doesn't mean dominant or passive as in the image of a doormat. It means you are Jesus-reliant and come before God with an honest heart and mind.

Identify & Interrogate negative or sinful thoughts you say to yourself. For example you say: "I never have fun at parties. No one is going to like me at this party." What if someone else said to you, "You never have fun at parties. No one is going to like you at this party. You better not come."

I hope you said that you'd dispute what they said—stand up for yourself. When we say these negative things to ourselves, we assume they are true. We generally have the skill of disputing other people when they make false accusations. We can learn to do so with ourselves as well.

Set your mind and heart on God. Paul taught, "Therefore we *do not lose heart.* Though outwardly we are wasting away, yet *inwardly* we are being *renewed* day by day ... So *we fix our eyes* not on what is seen, but on what is unseen" (2 Cor. 4:16–18, *my emphasis*). *It's not about me!*

Maybe you have been asking God *why* and are not getting any answers. It would not be unlike the devil to now be telling you that this book is a lie—that God doesn't care about your problems. He's not listening. He's absent. That is a lie! God Almighty is a mysterious God. We don't get all our questions answered. His thoughts and ways don't always line up with our thoughts or ways (Isa. 55:8). This is when we set our spirit towards only him and rest in our faith—in him alone!

Thank and Praise God. David sang: "I will praise God's name in song and glorify him with thanksgiving" (Ps. 69:30). When we give *thanks,* our focus is on what God has done for us. During *praise,* the focus is solely on him, his character, magnificence, and omniscience.

You should never have difficulty thinking of reasons why God deserves your thanks and praise. "The moment they began to sing and *to praise,* the Lord caused the armies of Ammon, Moab, and Mount Seir [*the bad guys*] to begin fighting among themselves, and *they destroyed each other!* (2 Chron. 20:22, TLB, *my emphasis*) ... Watch the devil run!

Part Three

Refocusing the Present and the Future

I, the LORD, speak the truth; I declare what is right.

—The Lord God, Isaiah 45:19

Perhaps it is good to have a beautiful mind. But an even greater gift is to discover a beautiful heart.

—John Nash, A Beautiful Mind

The Spirit gives life; the flesh counts for nothing. The words I have spoken to you are spirit and they are life.

—Jesus, John 6:63

Savior or Adversary?

All around us we witness the good, the bad, and the ugly in people and circumstances. We wonder why unrighteous people seem to prosper and the righteous suffer. Some people say if God is all-powerful, all-wise, and all-loving, he would eliminate the bad in the world.

Many question why God allows church leaders to devaluate the truth. Why does he tolerate deception to run rampant in his church, permitting disguised angels of light to infiltrate the body of Christ (2 Cor. 11:13–15)?

In 2005, Hurricane Katrina devastated New Orleans and the surrounding areas. It was defined by the insurance industry as an "Act of God." Called *natural evil,* many people believe disasters are acts of God, from birth defects to loss of babies, handicaps, disabilities, and violent deaths to wars, hurricanes, floods, droughts, plagues, and diseases of all sorts.

Natural evil does not involve human willing and acting but is still a result of the fall. In the aftermath of Katrina, one pastor was quoted saying God caused the hurricane as punishment for the sin that ran rampant in the city of New Orleans. Another pastor said God was merciful because most of the people got out of the city before a major levy broke.

A righteous, perfect God plus the existence of evil in the world does raise questions. Let's face it. God just doesn't perform up to our expectations. When you put your trust in God, you expect him to save you from evil. Most of us would agree that suffering and death are natural results of sin and, therefore, are not God's will any more than sin is. Even so, it too often appears the battle is turning in the enemy's favor.

If you have ever watched a wrestling match, it is usually not pretty. Wrestling means you get down and get dirty. There is no half-hearted involvement. You give it everything you've got or you lose. The winner usually attributes victory to knowing his opponent's moves and motives.

We are in a similar match with Satan, and we can even say with God. It's easy to admit we are in a daily wrestling match with Satan, but God?

The patriarch Jacob wrestled with God in Genesis 32:22–32. In their struggle, the man [*God*] said, "Let me go, for it is daybreak." Jacob replied, "I will not let you go unless you bless me."

The man [*God*] asked him, "What is your name?"

"Jacob," he answered. Then the man [*God*] said, "Your name will no longer be Jacob, but Israel, because you have struggled with God and with men and have overcome" (Gen. 26–28).

From the moment of our conversion, we are in an ongoing wrestling match of change. Satan's motive: to keep us in bondage. God's motive: to grow us into Christlikeness. There are moments when God must break our self-confidence in order that we submit to his plan and methods. Jacob finally surrenders and requests a blessing. God blesses him and changes his name to *Israel* to reflect the change in his character. *Israel* means "God strives" or "God rules."

God demonstrates his strength and perfect love in the midst of Jacob's weaknesses. God gave him a weakness as a reminder of his sovereignty (Gen. 32:25). Wrestling with God will bring victory when such struggling is done by means of prayer and earnestly seeking his favor.

Reflect: When was the last time you quit before receiving the blessing of God?

A Supernatural Wrestling Match

Jacob's wrestling match was a physical picture of his need for God. In all his previous human efforts to gain the blessing through deception, his real enemy had been God. Some of the wrestling matches with God reveal our selfish motives, rather than a desire for God's glory.

We may feel like we are in a supernatural wrestling match with God, but Scripture says, "neither angels nor demons, neither the present nor the future, nor any powers, neither height nor depth, nor any other created thing, will be able to separate us from the love of God, that is in Christ Jesus our Lord" (Rom. 8:38–39).

There is a story of a family who had a dog that had to be destroyed. The father said he'd do it himself. So he took the dog to a local river and threw him into the rapids. Mustering up all its strength, the dog swam against the current toward the father. As the dog got closer, the father threw a large stone at the dog, gashing the top of its head. Determined, the dog continued to swim toward the father. He took a large stick and kept hitting the dog with it, trying to throw him off balance so he would be swept away. Then the father fell in. The dog swam toward him, clamped onto him and pulled him to shore.

There is nothing we can do that is so bad he'd turn his back on us and leave us on Satan's doorstep. As intimidating as evil is, nothing you will ever face intimidates God. *He is so powerful he can direct any evil to a blessing.* He has seen it all and has already defeated every form of wickedness. Evil never catches him off guard like it does us.

Sometimes we have to get into a wrestling match before we are ready to receive the Father's mercy and grace. There are times when God knows the only way to get you where he wants to take you is to lead you down the path that passes through a dark valley. It's easy in that valley to only see the enemy, not God.

Instead of judging God through other people's words or worldly situations, we must get to know him, his moves and motives. We judge God by his Word. "God is light, and in him is no darkness at all" (1 John 1:5).

Mysteriously, God brings good and love from what seems like utter despair or evil. In his book, *Polishing God's Monuments*, pastor Jim Andrews wrote:

Sometimes in the mysteries of his wise providence, our heavenly Father finds it necessary to expose us to prickly hedges of disappointment, disaster, and despair. Whenever you find yourself among those thorns, expect the enemy to jump into your thinking like a dog on a bone ... Whenever we Christians take our place on the field of faith, we would be wise to prepare ourselves for this onslaught. Satan's subversive activity pursues our faith like a relentless knight ... Because Satan has been around the block, he knows that God, in the mystery of his purposes, will at intervals prescribe heavy burdens for his servants. During these times faith may stagger under the load ... Our adversary regularly waits in ambush for convenient crises that offer him the opportunity to invade our thinking ... There will be times when God seems to go on vacation and leaves us stranded in distress and despair without relief or prospect of deliverance. This, my friend, is the mystery side of God.[93]

Each moment of pain compels us to ask God very pointed questions, *Why did Mom die? Why did the man I love hurt me? In the mist of so much evil, are you really a good God?* These questions reveal not only a battle with Satan, with people and circumstances, but a battle with God.

Some Christians believe all suffering is from the devil. They blame Satan for every failure. When a leader commits adultery or embezzles money or abuses someone, often we hear, "The devil is working overtime." This response denies human dysfunction and the hand of God.

First, let's not omit the fact there is natural suffering simply because we are human. We cannot prevent the achy, aging process; or viruses from attacking, or losing loved ones. Being a fragile human in a dangerous, germy world cannot be blamed on the devil.

Second, we are each responsible for our behavior. Some of us simply leave the door wide open for Satan to walk in. Others have inherited a genetic disposition toward an illness, addiction, or other emotional disorders. Satan will take advantage of any physical and mental weak points, which is why it is important we understand our own biological and personality composition so we can cope positively.

I believe God allows, via our free will, humans to do their very worst as a result of the fall, yet still accomplish his purposes. The Bible clearly teaches that even fallen man has freedom of choice. We may not be of this world, but we live in it and are susceptible...but have an everlasting hope (see Rom. 8:18–23).

Lastly, recognize that what is often mistaken as a satanic attack may actually be God's hand of discipline upon us (Heb. 12:10). We will miss what God wants to do in our lives if we dismiss all suffering as Satan's doing.

Some Christians have difficulty with this truth because they cannot believe that a God of love could be responsible for either personal or public disasters. It may at times seem questionable, but never forget

Reflect: Satan will seek to plant the thoughts that God is angry with us and is disciplining us out of wrath. We fight back with the Word of God: "For when he punishes you, it proves that he loves you" (Heb. 12:6, TLB). God deals with me in perfect love." List three positive aspects to suffering.

The Battle of Job

We all battle these debilitating forces. Some of us come out transformed and victorious; some of us bruised and bloody. There are some things God can build into our lives only through suffering. We witness the same anguish as we read the book of Job.

Job's story brings us to the edge. It is a story of suffering and failure for which there is no explanation. It's the very worst things happening to the very best person at the hand of Satan. What is unique about the book of Job is in the first two chapters we get a glimpse of supernatural activity normally hidden from our view.

In chapter one, Satan asked God's permission to test Job.

God said Job was upright and blameless in his sight. Yet, God allowed Satan to test him. Now the scene was set to determine if Job would trust God in humanly impossible situations. He endured loss like few have known. His home was destroyed. His children died. His finances were wiped out. How does he react? Job fell to his knees, "The LORD gave and the LORD has taken away; may the name of the LORD be praised" (Job 1:20–21). Wow! I wonder how many parents that lost a child in a school shooting fell to the ground and worshipped God.

Satan proposes what seems like a contest to see if Job will remain a righteous man in suffering. God allows that challenge. God didn't cause it to happen, but he permitted it. The Bible says, "In all this, Job did not sin by charging God with wrong-doing." As tempting as it must have been, Job didn't scorn or revile God.

As you read Job and the psalms of David, these men give a piece of their minds and hearts to God, but they never blame him directly. In fact, as you read David's psalms, many begin in a voice of bitterness and depression, but then move to thanksgiving and praise for God. David chooses to get past his negative, toxic feelings. He chooses, in faith, to have confidence in God. He battles Satan with godly affirmation and rules!

We, too, should thank God for the trials. We may not enjoy the trial, but we can rejoice because we are in the will of God, and we know he is in control. Satan hates it when we thank and praise God.

In chapter two, just when Job didn't think it could get any worse, Satan came back—of course. He's got a new wager for God. Satan says anybody would give up on God if their health was taken away. God said he could test Job by making him sick, but he was not allowed to kill Job. Typical of the devil, he picks one of the most miserable sicknesses. He caused Job to be covered from head to foot with painful, pusy boils.

Job's wife wasn't handling this very well. "Are you still holding on to your integrity? Curse God and die!" (Job 2:9). I think she gets a bum rap. She just lost all her children! Who knows what we may say in such a situation. Loss draws out those toxic emotions.

There appears to be a boxing match between God and Satan often coined the "The Duel." While we must not ignore the reality of spiritual warfare, we must remember that the contest is not between equals. God is always sovereign (Job 1:12). Satan is on a chain under God's authority and control.

Reflect: God may not change your circumstances, but he can change your mind so the circumstances will work for you and not against you. How might God be doing that now in your life?

Our Emotions Reveal Our Perceptions

For Job, the facts didn't add up. He did nothing to deserve these calamities. He moves through a range of emotions, much like we would. He grieves. He's depressed. He wishes he were dead. We watch Job getting angrier, which is normal because anger accompanies grief. Job paints God as a villain, "God assails me and tears me in his anger and gnashes his teeth at me. Though I cry, 'I've been wronged!' I get no response; though I call for help, there is no justice" (Job 16:9; 19:7).

These are feelings of entrapment and angst. Job is a tormented man. Feelings are complex and often based on potent past memories. We can understand why Job was bitter, what awful memories he carried in his mind each day.

What we don't usually realize is our feelings sometimes lie. Like Job, many people believe their feelings without proving them. For example: "*I feel* like you don't love me." "*I feel* stupid, like a failure." "*I feel* you can't ever trust me again." We have to place our confidence on God's promises, his Word, and not our feelings. His Word is 100 percent reliable! Our feelings are manipulated by circumstances, other people, and hormones and past experiences. Whereas, God is a promise keeper. We can cling to his promises. Even better—we can rest in them. They will never fail.

Whenever you have a strong negative feeling, check it against God's Word. For example, if you are angry, look up verses and passages that speak to anger. Then ask, "Do I have a valid reason to feel mad?" or is the bitterness coming from stuffed feelings from a past event? Job certainly had a reason to feel angry.

Had God really abandoned him? No. As soon as God spoke to Job, he recognized he should not have challenged God's wisdom, and he turns the corner. "I know that you can do all things; no plan of yours can be thwarted" (Job 42:2). Job's perception of the situation changed. He finally beheld God's unfathomable greatness in his circumstances. He came to understand God was infinitely wiser than he (Job 42:1–4).

Although demons cannot inhabit believers, God sometimes permits Satan to afflict Christians with adversity. Dr. Warren Wiersbe said, "When God permits Satan to light the furnace, he always keeps his own hand on the thermostat!"[94] Satan cannot defeat the person who trusts in God.

Erik Weihenmayer, the first blind person to climb Mount Everest said, "You don't just deal with adversity. You use it to propel you forward."[95] Don't resent the hardships. God did not spare his own Son. God will reveal his character to you in ways you never knew. You will see him more clearly as he takes you through the dark times.

In the final chapter, Job has come to know God. God lifts Job up, blesses him, and restores everything twofold because that is God's nature: to free us and restore joy. Job's wife survives and bears ten more children. I wonder if Job realized his experience brought glory to God in the face of this cosmic struggle?

Job never witnessed Christ's presence, but he had that future hope. He exclaimed, "I know that my Redeemer lives" (Job 19:25). [In ancient Israel, a redeemer bought a slave's way to freedom or took care of a widow.]

What incredible faith Job had, especially in light of the fact he was unaware of the discussion between God and Satan. Job is an example of a man deeply tested—not punished—by God. Job never believed he was no good because of his affliction. If affliction is allowed, it is to do some extraordinary work.

There are some secrets God has chosen not to reveal (Deut. 29:29; 1 Cor. 2:16). God is infinite and all-knowing. His motivations and purposes are beyond our reach. God keeps us ignorant because we just can't understand his supernatural view from above.

It is in the darkness of our emotional wrestling with God that we grow in our understanding of him. Recognize your trial may be yet another way God is working transformation by bringing into your life circumstances that are designed to cause you to grow spiritually. We say, "If it's possible, Lord, may I see your reason for this trial? I know it's not to hurt me."

Each of us was given the gift of free will. We have a choice to make everyday: to call on God for supernatural help and submit, or leave the door open for Satan's crew to begin construction on a new mindhold.

Nothing happens without God's direction or permission. His sovereignty directs every situation to accomplish his purposes, causing adversity to work together for good. What is encouraging to me is God is working simultaneously with the evil efforts of sinful human beings and Satan. These evil efforts become the very means of accomplishing his purposes.

Romans 8:28 gives us encouragement, "We know that in all things God works for the good of those who love him, who have been called according to his purpose." Paul is actually talking about our spiritual transformation. The "good" of verse 28 is explained in verse 29: "For those God foreknew he also predestined to be conformed to the likeness of his Son." He uses every circumstance in some mysterious way to transform us more into the likeness of his Son (2 Cor. 3:18). "He who began a good work in you will carry it on" (Phil. 1:6). We are all unfinished projects to God.

Reflect: How does this story help you understand God's activity in your life now?

A Thorn in the Flesh

A well-known passage is James 1:2–5. When we are suffering in life we need to ask God for wisdom to understand and profit by it. Sometimes, the answer returns, "I am allowing you to suffer in order to draw you closer to me. I am letting you hurt in order to heal you at a deeper level." The Apostle Paul had this experience.

In order to keep Paul from being prideful and boastful, God permitted Satan to afflict Paul. He expresses his battle with God, "To keep me from becoming conceited there was given me a thorn in my flesh, a messenger of Satan, to torment me. Three times I pleaded with the Lord to take it away from me. But he said to me, 'My grace is sufficient for you, for my power is made perfect in weakness'" (2 Cor. 12:7–9).

Paul wrote of a spiritual experience where he saw sights and sounds that a mortal should not experience. An encounter like this could have filled him with overwhelming pride, which, in turn, would have completely destroyed his walk with God and the effectiveness of his ministry.

Theologians have debated repeatedly what Paul's thorn was. Tradition has taught that Paul's thorn in the flesh was some type of physical ailment or sickness. The focus in these verses is on Paul's weakness and God's all sufficient grace, not the thorn itself. He asked God for deliverance from a specific weakness three times.

God's first response to Paul's pleading for the removal of his thorn was no. Recall Jesus prayed three times in the Garden of Gethsemane that the cup might pass from him, and God said no. God's second response to Paul was "My grace is sufficient for you." I imagine their conversation went something like this:

Paul said, "But Lord ..."

God said, "I've given you sufficient grace, which will be more than enough for whatever you face."

Paul replies, "Why, Lord?"

"Because my power is perfected in your weakness."

"Lord, power is perfected in success. That makes us strong—achievement."

"No. Achievement makes you proud. Thorns make you weak and when you are weak you are humble and I receive the glory."

Paul wanted to increase his power by the removal of the thorn. In order for Paul to grow spiritually, he would need to admit he couldn't do everything on his own. To gain spiritual strength, he would have to be weak first, at least in his thinking.

His affliction had to meet grace in order to bring about its God-intended result. Power came through seeing weakness as the very vehicle for manifesting the power of Christ. Only in his weakness did Paul trust implicitly in God. God did not answer Paul's prayer, but he met Paul's needs.

There is not one of us who does not have some kind of a thorn in the flesh. It may be a personal weakness, handicap, unhappy marriage or employment, or financial hardship. God gets our attention through these thorns. As with Paul, some thorns may never go away, but God's grace is sufficient to handle them for life.

Clearly Satan does not give us adversity to keep us from becoming conceited—just the opposite. This passage attributes "a messenger of Satan" as something given with God's intention for our good and his glory. Very rarely do we find pride in people who have been broken apart in anguish and pain. There is no pride when you find out your husband has been cheating on you. There is no pride when your dream has been shelved over and over again or when your teenager publicly defies you. Only humility.

When I was told by a high-profile ministry I would be one of their featured speakers, I was ecstatic. For months I prayed God would bless this opportunity and remove all obstacles Satan might throw in the way. Then I learned the feature was going to be delayed, possibly cancelled, not once, but twice. This news became my "messenger of Satan." I had to discern whether the devil was victorious in delaying this project or whether God was the one who put up the obstacles because it wasn't the right time. Or perhaps I simply wasn't ready for this kind of exposure.

Reflect and pray: Almighty God, I praise you for sharing your grace and your strength—through Jesus—with me that I might glorify you with my life!

The Answer is No

Paul demonstrates that we do have the right to pray for healing from illness. Prayer aligns our life with God but at times he does say no to our prayers. Paul was not healed. The purpose of prayer is not to conform God to our will but to adjust our will to God's. Have you ever thought what might happen if all your prayers were answered? When we pray, we have to ask ourselves, "Does this request bring glory to Jesus or me"?

Mother Teresa said more tears are shed over answered prayers than unanswered prayers. Garth Brooks sang, "Sometimes I thank God for unanswered prayers. Remember when you're talkin' to the man upstairs that just because he doesn't answer doesn't mean he don't care" (Lyrics: "Unanswered Prayers"[96]).

Paul's failure to be healed didn't devastate him. On the contrary, it enhanced his ministry. When God allows sickness or sorrow into our lives, we are tempted to question his wisdom. Often we ask "Why, Lord?" God is under no obligation to answer us or make us prosperous. Whether our circumstances are easy or difficult, we can completely trust God's wisdom. "I will take delight in my people; the sound of weeping and of crying will be heard in it [Jerusalem] no more" (Isa. 65:19).

Termed "the dark night of the soul," great believers have, and still do today, experienced bouts of agonizing doubt in their God. In Robert Kelleman's book, *Beyond the Suffering*. Nellie, a former slave from Savannah, Georgia says, "It has been a terrible mystery, to know why the good Lord should so long afflict my people, and keep them in bondage—to be abused, and trampled down, without any rights of their own—with no ray of light in the future. Some of my folks said there wasn't any God, for if there was He wouldn't let white folks do as they have done for so many years."

A slave, Polly, responds and embraces hope, "We poor creatures have need to believe in God, for if God Almighty will not be good to us some day, why were we born? When I heard of his delivering his people from bondage I know it means the poor Africans."[97]

God has promised to bless us; but those blessings are often more spiritual than physical. In those difficult or questionable times, God says, "Just watch what I am going to do!" He knows what is best for us. That is love.

Reflect on Nellie's perspective, and then Polly's. Then read Psalms 103, a psalm of praise. Meditate on David's words about our amazing God.

R.E.S.I.S.T. Recap

Recognize all suffering is not from the devil and that you are responsible for your response and ultimately your behavior. Your trial may be another way God is working transformation by bringing into your life circumstances that are designed to cause you to grow spiritually.

Embrace God's hand of discipline upon you or any agonizing doubts about God. There are some things God can build into your life only through suffering and questioning. How willing are you to embrace distress for the sake of God's will?

Submit if you find yourself in a wrestling match with God. You won't win! It may be God's way of telling you that he has a different plan for your life and that you need him. He will get the glory for your changed life.

Identify & Interrogate any strong negative feeling and then check it against God's Word. For example, if you are angry, look up verses and passages that speak to anger. Do you have a valid reason to feel mad? Trust and rest in God alone.

Set your mind and heart on God even though he may not change your circumstances. If you are battling with God today, put your painful feelings into words and on paper. *Lord, may I see your reason for this trial?*

Thank and Praise God for trials. He walks closely with you even if all you can see is the enemy. Praise him for working to bring good and love from what seems like utter despair or evil. You may not enjoy the trial, but you can rejoice because you are in the will of God. He is in control!

Embracing Your Personality

When I say the word *authenticity,* what comes to mind? We believe we need to camouflage our imperfections and problems. We think, *I'll be likeable, accepted and hopefully admired if I give the impression I'm perfect.* Most women learned early in life to conceal their shortcomings and wear a mask. Many of us have become pros at masking the problems and the pain. This concealment requires a great deal of energy. It may even destroy us, as it did me.

Cover Girl masks are toxic and pure poison to our relationships. We can become independent, believing we can manage life on our own. *I don't need anybody else!* We can isolate. We can become the super-mom or the super-businesswoman, too busy to let anyone else inside our life.

The task of breaking down mindholds requires breaking our masks completely. We all experience tension between the masked self and the true self—between the flesh and the spirit. The true self is the image of God within us, the part of us made in the likeness of God. The masked self is the constructed image we've created to deal with the world. It is defensive and self-protective. It is our selfish side that makes intimacy with God and others difficult. Jesus calls us to deny our masked selves so we can authentically follow him.

The Pharisees brought a woman caught in adultery and placed her out in front of the crowd (John 8:3–11). Moses's law said to stone her to death. Jesus stood up and said, "All right, hurl the stones at her until she dies. But only he who never sinned may throw the first!" The Jewish leaders slipped away one by one until only Jesus was left in front of the crowd with the woman.

The Pharisees were exposed for who they really were, their masks torn off by Jesus. Then Jesus stood up again and said to her, "Where are your accusers? Didn't even one of them condemn you?" "No, sir," she said. Jesus said, "Neither do I. Go and sin no more." Her mask was discarded.

We want to learn to embrace and love our true self intimately and put aside the masked self. When I acknowledge I am a new person in Jesus Christ, I accept that old things, including past traumas and emotional hurts, have passed away. I embrace that no matter what has happened that I am awesome and I enjoy life. *I am stamped in God's image!* We pray: "Jesus, tear off my mask so my true self is exposed!"

"Love takes off masks that we fear we cannot live without and know we cannot live within" (James Baldwin).[98] Jesus shows us what it means to know love, grace, and truth in him. Her real self didn't have to die for her sin or be separated from her Savior.

Reflect on this statement: What really matters is what happens *in us,* not to us.

The Image of God (*Imago Dei*)

God created us in his image and without a mask! Today when we hear the word *image,* it connotes something different than the likeness of God. An actress or politician hires an image manager. An executive dresses for success, conveying an image. A company seeks the right image.

How can we, fallen human beings, articulate the image of God? By virtue of being human, one is in the image of God. The image of God has not been lost as a result of sin or the fall. Even after the fall, murder was prohibited because human beings were made in the image of God (Gen. 9:6).

The image refers to all the elements in our makeup that enable the fulfillment of our destiny. It makes us, like God, capable of interacting with other persons, of thinking and acting, and using our God-given will freely.

Man's self-image thrives on physical attractiveness, athletic ability, or a place on the corporate ladder. When we approach Scripture, we encounter a new kind of image. Mother Teresa said that when she looked into the face of a dying beggar she prayed to see the face of Jesus so she might serve the beggar as she would serve Christ.[99]

Jesus, in the Sermon on the Mount (Matthew 5 and 6), blesses the poor, the grieving, the meek, the persecuted. He comments on how difficult it is for the rich to enter the kingdom of heaven. He condemns pride and self-sufficiency. In effect, he is said, "Fine-tune all your interests until the attitude of your mind and heart and body are on me."

As the Spirit works within us, we become more like him (2 Cor. 3:18), bearing his image. As a believer, "we have the amazing ability and the awesome responsibility to make visible the invisible attributes of the Creator and Redeemer" (Dr. Gerry Breshears).[100]

What we must decide is how we are valuable rather than how valuable we appear; *how we are authentic* rather than how authentic we appear. Are we going to be an image manager or an image bearer? "Certainly what one is, is of far greater importance than what one appears to be" (Emily Post).[101]

Paul, in speaking about Christian authenticity, said it is characterized by repentance, service, and waiting on the Lord (1 Thess. 1: 8–10). You have been placed on this earth as God's sovereign emblem, his representative. We reflect God when we love and forgive one another. The way you have been created is part of God's master plan which makes you a real and authentic person.

Understand the person you are today is determined by several factors: brain function, family of origin, modeling behavior after others, cultural influences, past and present circumstances, and memories. If we can begin to understand how we are put together, we will have a better understanding of our selves, how particular mindholds are constructed and deconstructed, and we are able to be image bearers.

Reflect: If you've gotten this far, I assume God has revealed a great deal to you about yourself. Where are you in the process of breaking your Cover Girl Mask? How do now understand yourself better? How are you a more authentic person today?

Personality Roles

We all begin life hardwired with a soul. As life unfolds, we collect psychological data in the form of experiences (a process that starts in the womb). As we absorb experiences, they are transformed into memories, which shape our learned responses, which, in turn, affect what we make of new experiences. We see this when young babies and their mothers interact. Recall, bonding with our mother during our first year determines how secure or insecure we will be.

As we grow up our personality starts to take form and we develop multiple roles over time. I start as a child creating roles in response to my relationship with my parents and my birth order. I form new roles as I begin to interact and relate in school and move forward with life. Today my roles are wife, daughter, women's pastor, step-grandmother, friend, sister, and God's daughter. I act differently depending on what role I'm playing.

The ability to play roles is part of the normal person's ability for relating with others. Jesus had different personality roles. One moment he is lambasting the Pharisees with words intended to break their hardened hearts, then we see him comforting a child, and the next minute he is lovingly disciplining and teaching an adulterous woman.

When I first encounter the heavenly Father, I may try to relate to him through one of my existing roles, often the one formed in response to my earthly father—the daughter role. Some of us come into a new relationship with God and have a flawed image or expectation of him.

One reason we hold false perceptions of God is our tendency to project onto God the unloving characteristics of the people we look up to, who is usually our earthly dad. If my dad abused me in any form, then God most likely is demanding or angry or remote. It will be hard for me to relate to God lovingly.

Our relationship with God also depends on brain function. If our brain is working right, we are more likely to see God as kind and loving. If our brain is overactive, we tend to color the world in a negative way, so we may see God as a judge and unloving.[102] We must develop our image of God from the Bible, not from false teachers or painful relationships.

The roles we develop are in response to other people (usually our parents) who have expectations for us and reward specific behaviors. If the expectations were not met, we were punished in some way. Then we develop a role that will exist in conflict, like the perfectionist, performer, or the victim.

My father has a powerful choleric temperament (meaning self-confident, likes to be in control and make all the decisions). To please him, a leading role emerged—the compliant, people-pleaser, which I'll call Role A. I also lived in several communities where women were defined by their perfected Cover Girl mask. In order to be accepted another role emerged, Role B—the (perceived) perfect Kimberly. Unconsciously, I fought against these roles so I created a new role, my rebel, suppressed role, Role C.

When Role C, gets out, it rebels because it's impossible to maintain the people-pleaser, perfect Cover Girl mask. It binges on food and alcohol and likes to party, because it doesn't get what it's seeking. Once the toxic episode subsides, the rebellious woman feels guilty and ashamed and retreats. Role A, the dominant survival personality, then comes out.

Personality roles change to cope with different situations. Even my husband has a different personality role when he is around my dad. When he feels confronted, a new role emerges— one I don't particularly like. As he puts it, it's his "survival-male" role. (By the way, I love my dad. He's a wonderful man.) Most of us have developed a survival personality, a Cover Girl mask, which makes us feel in control.

Our primary role may change suddenly. A daughter may have to take on the primary role of mother if her mother dies or becomes incapacitated. Talk about super-sizing your emotions! Life is constantly distracting and pressing our buttons, usually when we least expect it.

Are you beginning to understand why you do what you do?

We are also made up of all of our memories and life experiences that are responsible for our sense of identity and the way we interact with others. Personally, my memory bank contains a lot of data labeled "rejection" which causes me unconsciously to put up walls.

What I never realized is that these walls gave me an illusion of safety. What they really did was prevent me from getting what I needed to become whole. And then a personality test revealed I am 48% introvert. *It's okay to put people off. That's my personality!* Yes and no.

Introverts tend to be low-key, deliberate, and relatively less engaged in social situations. They are energized when alone. However, too often, parents or peers or co-workers try to push the introvert to socialize which often makes her feel like a fish out of water, like a so-called reject.

Acknowledging that introversion and extraversion are normal variants of behavior can help in self-acceptance and understanding ourselves and others. My behavior now makes sense to me. Now I choose to make the extra effort to connect and break down walls, which isn't always comfortable or easy. Effort is only effort when it starts to hurt. Jesus taught me that humans are relational. To him, spiritual health is what happens when relationships are intact. Sin is what happens when relationships are broken.

Reflect: Assess and compare your different personality roles. What is your primary personality role? Is one a survival type of personality role? Explain.

Our Role in Christ

The Bible says once Jesus Christ is our Savior, we become his daughter or son. You could say he is born into our mortal flesh. Think about that! Jesus said, "I have given them the glory that you [the Father] gave me, that they may be one as we are one: I in them and you in me" (John 17:22–23, my emphasis).

Kimberly Davidson

The Trinity takes up permanent residence inside of us. The Trinity means that God is one being who exists, simultaneously and eternally, as three persons: the Father, God; the Son, incarnate as Jesus of Nazareth; and the Holy Spirit. Each person is in us permanently, not for just a visit.

This is powerful because imagine, now, the Trinity is between not only you and Satan, but each person you have a relationship with. They are the power behind taking every toxic thought captive. That negative thought can now be tossed out by God himself. If I tend to bite and devour you each time our paths cross, I recognize if I hand off my anger to God, I will not verbally vomit all over you. If I tend to be a needy person, if I give God my needs and insecurities, I can be a more valuable friend. My mask breaks.

Secondly, when I am born-again, my heavenly Father calls me into relationship with him. I have a new role as God's daughter. This new part of my personality is "born of the Spirit" (John 3:8). My old life was centered around myself and hiding my problems. There is a new me existing in intimacy with the newly indwelling Spirit of God (1 John 4:13–15).

I am a new creation because Jesus lives in me (John 14:20). God himself is now working in me. That takes the pressure off us. God is now our image manager. But, we still have to do something: submit in complete dependence so the Holy Spirit can do his work. When we do we find God putting us in places and situations we never dreamed of.

The whole truth of our identification and image is achieved when we set our entire heart and mind on Christ. "For you have become a part of him, and so you died with him, so to speak, when he died; and now you share his new life and shall rise as he did. Your old evil desires were nailed to the cross with him; that part of you that loves to sin was crushed and fatally wounded, so that your sin-loving body is no longer under sin's control" (Rom. 6:5–6, TLB).

This is our Cinderella story. We no longer need to be a slave to sin and toxic thinking. As our mind grasps this truth, we really live because he lives in us. It's like a holy pregnancy. God's seed is implanted in our spirit (1 John 3:9). We are linked to Jesus by a holy umbilical cord, and beauty resonates from our inner self, which is of great worth in God's eyes (1 Pet. 3:3–4).

Reflect: If Jesus came to live in your home, how would you act? Would you put yourself down or gossip or play the comparison game?

It makes sense that if Jesus abides in me, I have no reason to put myself down, because now I'm putting him down. If I look in the mirror and say, "I'm so ugly," first, I'm telling God he made a mistake. Second, I'm pretty sure I'm calling him ugly now! All of a sudden our thoughts and actions take on a whole new meaning when he lives within us—within our home, his temple. Reflect on that.

The Dark Side

In the 1950s and 1960s, Mother Teresa wrote several letters, which were revealed after her death, to her church spiritual guides. The letters disclosed troubling and painful conflicts she sometimes had with her faith. At times, she even doubted the existence of God.

"I am told God lives in me—and yet the reality of darkness and coldness and emptiness is so great that nothing touches my soul," she wrote in one of the letters.

Some of the letters depict a spiritually bereft Teresa, struggling to maintain her belief. "Where I try to raise my thoughts to heaven, there is such convicting emptiness that those very thoughts return like sharp knives and hurt my very soul. Love— the word—it brings nothing," wrote the woman known as the "Messiah of Love."

Mother Teresa even struggled with depression. In another letter, Mother Teresa wrote, "In my soul, I can't tell you how dark it is, how painful, how terrible—I feel like refusing God."[103] When you wrestle with both God and Satan, and are surrounded by human misery, you have a reason to be depressed.

Open your mind and heart to the possibility that God is gently opening doors to the darker areas of your heart—those secret and ignored areas. The process of breaking mindholds and spiritual growth requires following the Spirit into our dark side and letting his light shine in.

As we have learned, we each have the capacity for both good and evil. It is the choice of each individual to determine which inclination will be most prominent. Jesus said, "The good man brings good things out of the good stored up in him, and the evil man brings evil things out of the evil stored up in him" (Matt. 12:35).

Dr. Les Carter said, "In order to keep the dark side of the personality from dominating, it is necessary to keep a constant vigil over it, lest it creep up and overtake much of our decision making."[104] If we have a dark area in our heart that needs to be exposed, we must allow the Holy Spirit to cleanse our heart at its source.

What negative traits play out in the story of your life? Every person has some sort of personal dysfunction. "Mostly, our souls are shadowed places; we live at the border where our dark side blocks our light and throws a shadow over our interior places ... We cannot always tell where our light ends and our shadow begins or where our shadow ends and our darkness begins" (Lewis Smedes).[105]

Toxic emotions such as self-absorption, anger, fear, lust, anxiety, and jealousy, to name the most common, come out of our dark side. Those who deny or are unaware of their dark side have a bull's-eye on their back. We have all witnessed high-profile evangelical leaders who have been brought down by their dark side. The authors of *Overcoming the Dark Side of Leadership* reveal:

Many in the Christian community relegate the problem [fallen spiritual leaders] entirely to the realm of spiritual warfare and demonic attack. But the problem is not that easily dismissed ... America and the church discovered a generation plagued by a plethora of personal dysfunctions: codependence, addictive behaviors, obsessive-compulsive disorders, narcissistic personality disorder, paranoia, codependence, passive-aggressive behavior, or any one of a host of others.

At times the dark side seems to leap on us unexpectedly. In reality it has slowly crept up on us. The development of our dark side has been a lifetime in the making despite the fact the assault by these powerful emotions, compulsions, and dysfunctions can be sudden. Like vinegar and soda being slowly swirled together in a tightly closed container, our personalities have been slowly intermingled with emotions, expectations, and experiences that over time have created our dark side. If not tended, the mixture will ultimately explode with great ferocity.[106]

Reflect: Take some time to look past your actions to what lies behind them. Ask God to help you see what he sees when he examines your motives. "Lord, show me what is in my heart. Why did I do this [*addiction, lies, premarital sex, shoplift, gossip, abortion, affair*]? Reveal to me how my behaviors made me feel back then. How are they affecting me today? Show me why I created a destructive pattern and how I've become deceived and distorted your truth." This is mind interrogation.

Embracing Our Dark Side

In *The Screwtape Letters*, the veteran demon Screwtape instructs Wormwood, "You must bring him [her] to a condition in which he [she] can practice self-examination for an hour *without discovering any of those facts about himself* which are perfectly clear to anyone who's ever lived in the same house with him or worked in the same office."[107]

This is Satan's objective: to get us to believe interrogation is unproductive or too painful. We believe the lie and resort to various coping mechanisms that simply cover up the problem instead of addressing it. Self-examination is a light shedding process—the light of truth penetrates and exposes the dark side of deception.

The truth is many of our emotions are like unwanted company or extended family. We're stuck with them. We can fight them, mask them, deny them, or stuff them away until they eat wreak havoc in our bodies and lives. Or, we can acknowledge they exist, learn to embrace and manage them before the damage is done.

Sue Grafton studies the dark side of people. She wrote in *USA Weekend,* "We all need to look into the dark side of our nature—that's where the energy is, the passion. People are afraid of it because it holds pieces of us we're busy denying."[108]

We must discover and redeem our dark side in order to win our personal battles. Justifying, denying, or blaming only intensifies the war. The battle may not directly involve or be caused by Satan. Certainly, his motive is to keep us in denial that we even have a dark side.

Through this process I learned I have a perfectionist or obsessive-compulsive nature. As a child of this world I channeled that energy into my appearance, and subsequently an eating disorder. Today, as a child of God, I still have that disposition. The difference is I submit it to God, channeling that energy into something productive for the Kingdom, like this book!

If I become too obsessive with my writing, physically, I get knots in my neck. My head and my right hand and elbow begin to ache. My shoulders become tight and my sitting muscles strained. I recognize this, so I take frequent breaks.

Spiritually, becoming obsessive about anything has the potential to get in the way of my relationship with God—even if it is a good thing, like writing this book. You may become obsessive about something as innocent as bike riding. If riding detracts you from God, it becomes idolatry and is sin in God's eyes.

Recognizing you have a dark side and embracing it is a giant step to breaking your mask and living in freedom. Embracing means we stop blaming the devil, our parents, our circumstances, culture, and others. The truth is our dark side can be a blessing in disguise.

> We wonder if we're capable of doing anything with pure motives. We languish under the powerful grip of unhealthy attitudes, behaviors, and habits that have been a lifetime in the making and we are led to the brink of despair. This is exactly the gift our dark side offers. When it is completely acknowledged, free of rationalization and excuses, we will either throw our hands up in despair or be driven to cry out for God's grace in recognition of our total dependence on him (Gary McIntosh and Samuel Rima, Sr.).[109]

Reflect: Briefly describe what you think your dark side is. Begin to examine and interrogate the condition of your relationships. Maybe it's anger in the form of abuse, depression, or ongoing negative thoughts. It might be addiction or low-self esteem. What lies and wounds have surfaced? What accusations do you wear as your identity? What temptations are you continually enslaved to? Let the light of Jesus in on these areas.

I would also suggest you take a personality profile test and study the four main personality types (choleric, sanguine, melancholy, phlegmatic). Learn about your birth order. While temperaments describe who we are, birth order helps explain why we've become that way. The order in which we were born into our family shapes our personality in deep-seated ways. You can find this information online. There are many books that can help you discover your dark side and develop your divine design.

Dark Thinking—Light Thinking

With a lump in her throat, Jenny confided to her Bible study group, "When I am at work and around other people, like my family and friends, I control what I am eating. A lot of the time I don't even think about having seconds…or thirds. But when I get home and I'm all alone, that's when I lose control. I'll sit for hours, numb, eating junk food. Why can I control my eating around other people, but not around myself?"

Jenny openly confessed her battle with food. This was the starting point to breaking this mindhold. She asked *why*. Some people advise that you tell your negative thought or emotion, "Go away. Just give it to God and let him take care of it. Don't dwell on it." As Dr. Phil says, "How has that worked for you?"

To receive God's power over your dark side, first, acknowledge its existence in your life and recognize God's empowering work through it. Praise him for that! Second, make a commitment to understand the shape it has taken in your life by examining and interrogating your thoughts regularly. A problem cannot be solved until it is honestly faced and opened up. We won't get the results we want until we take ownership for our attitudes. To merely send your thought away is to leave an opening for another thought dart to take hold. Rather, interrogate it! *Reveal the why, Lord!*

When prisoners are taken captive, they are interrogated. When we take a thought captive, we do the same: "*Why* am I thinking this way?" We ask God for information. "*Why* am I feeling so fearful and rejected today? This is the third time this week!" Don't be afraid to go down the narrow path.

We ask God, "Why do I keep doing what I don't want to do? Keep sinning? Where is this coming from?" God began to reveal to Jenny the source of her battle with food. She couldn't stand to be by herself. It actually terrified her. So she ate. The fear came from the fact her dad left her and her mom when she was three years old.

The source of this mindhold was exposed and Jenny had a choice to make. Either, *in faith*, she could get to the source of her feelings of abandonment and inability to be alone. Or, *in fear*, leave the wound alone and live in pain and denial, eating herself to death. If she follows her faith-based emotions, God will begin peeling the onion layers away, possibly through counseling and pastoral intervention.

We're now beginning to get into the habit of taking every thought captive in obedience to Christ. This means asking the Holy Spirit to clarify whether that thought will help me or hurt me. Taking a thought captive goes one of two ways. If it is a non-repetitive toxic thought such as *I wish I had her success*, I reject it and give it to Jesus. I may reason: *With every successful job come headaches.*

However, if with every woman I see I think, *I wish I had her success*, I want to confront that thought and find out why I keep thinking this way. "Lord, what is it that I am seeking? What has created this void?"

Once I started interrogating my thoughts and actions versus blowing them off, as in just get over it, God was able to expose and clean out a lot of old junk and hurts. Embracing and overcoming our dark side means we get into the habit of interrogating where the toxic thought comes from.

Many women fear confronting the memories of the past. Why do we need to? To know *the why* opens the door to seeing the possibility of seeing the seriousness of a problem and the need for more than "Just stop" or "Go away thought." Often mere behavior modification isn't the answer. Recognition of the motivation behind the thought or behavior reveals our need to avail ourselves to the work of the Holy Spirit so he can expose the darkness and bring truth and light into our life.

When we understand the memory or the thought, the soul heals because we are freed from unnecessary guilt, anxiety, and shame. The memory that was buried alive is released. We claim our identity as God's daughter and move toward permanent Christlikeness. Satan has no more power. Denial disappears. Mask broken! Interrogation is to embrace God's biblical path for your life. With the guidance of the Holy Spirit, ask:

1. What is the source? Where did that thought come from? The devil, the flesh, or the world? Yes! Toss it out.

2. Can I defend this thought from the Word of God? No! Toss it out.

3. Is this pride? Is this about me receiving credit? Am I thinking too highly of myself or poorly about someone else? Yes! Toss it out.

4. If I follow this thought will this get me where God wants me to go in life? No! Toss it out.

5. Will this thought build me up or tear me down? Jealousy, greed, anger, and pride will tear you down. Toss it out.

6. Will I reap freedom and joy by allowing this thought through my sieve? No! Toss it out.

7. Is this thought scripturally sound? Is it truth? *Go ahead and do it … everybody's doing it.* No! Toss it out.

8. Can I share this thought? No! Toss it out.

9. Does this thought make me feel shamed or condemned? Yes! Toss it out.

10. Does this fit who I am (my character) as the daughter and a follower of Jesus? No! Toss it out.

11. Does this thought bring glory to Jesus? No! Toss it out.

12. Am I buying into the devil's message through romance novels, soap operas, gossipy conversations, movies, or magazines? Yes! Toss it out.

Reflect: God's Word says, "It is for freedom that Christ has set us free. Stand firm, then, and do not let yourselves be burdened again by a yoke of slavery" (Gal. 5:1). Stand firm on your foundation of who God is. Stand firm on who you are in Jesus Christ. Stand firm on your faith on all of God's promises every day.

Pray: Jesus, thank you for continuing to liberate me. Your word says you have rescued me out of the darkness and gloom of Satan's kingdom and brought me into your kingdom of light.

You bought my freedom with your blood and forgave all my sins—past, present, and future (Col. 1:13–14). Deliver me today from any yoke of bondage by revealing anything that needs to be broken and restored by you. Help me to recognize and stand strong against my enemies and stand firm in who I am in you.

R.E.S.I.S.T. Recap

Recognize there is an ongoing symphony of tension between your Cover Girl false self and your true self—between your flesh and the spirit.

Embrace that no matter what has happened, you are awesome. Say, "I am stamped in God's image! God sees me as perfect and accepts me exactly the way I am now."

Submit to the Holy Spirit's leading so he can do his work, creating your new role as God's daughter while tossing out old thinking. Submit the fear of confronting the memories of the past. What are the thoughts and fears no one hears but you?

Identify & Interrogate—The process of breaking mindholds and continued growth into Christlikeness requires identifying your dark side. God may be opening the doors to the darker areas of your heart and mind. Are you beginning to become aware of the ways your negative traits play out in your life today?

Set your mind and heart on God as you open up your mind to what lies behind your past actions. What do you think your dark side is? What lies and wounds have surfaced? What accusations do you wear as your identity? What temptations are you continually enslaved to?

Thank and Praise God for the personality—characteristics, flaws, and temperament, he gave you. Thank him that your dark side can be a blessing in disguise. Praise him for continuing to liberate and deliver you from the yoke of bondage by revealing what needs to be broken and restored.

Losing Your (Old) Mind

More than six million adolescents mutilate themselves with razors, glass, knives, and nails. Jordan cut herself over two hundred times within the last year. Maria has been pulling out her hair, eyebrows, and lashes for at least ten years. She told her mom that she really hates what she does to herself, that she tries to stop, but she can't help herself.

Cutting or self-abuse may be an extreme, but we all have a fleshly fight on our hands. Maybe it's gossip or lack of self-control over sweets or impatience with our extended family. It's like our angel and the devil are battling it out on a daily, and sometimes, on a minute-by-minute basis.

Paul, too, felt tormented. "I do not understand what I do. For what I want to do I do not do, but what I hate I do" (Rom. 7:15). Paul speaks as one caught helplessly between a desire for good and a rebellious will. Paul felt the inner tensions between his own personality roles. Paul the Pharisee is at war with Paul the Christian.

His solution was a relationship with God (as defined in Romans 8). His relationship with God did not solve the inner tensions. The war still ensued, but the nature of the struggle changed. When the Holy Spirit came to live within Paul and took up his role as counselor, guide, companion, the Spirit had a fight on his hands—a fight with the old Paul, the Pharisee.

"Little does he [Paul] know how healthy his condition is, and this shattering discovery is but the prelude to a magnificent series of further discoveries of things which God has expressly designed for his eternal enrichment" (Miles J. Stanford).[110] I believe Christians often feel uncomfortable admitting to pessimistic thinking or addictive behavior because we mistakenly believe our faith should eliminate all our problems.

The fact is our new self and our new mind (guided by the Holy Spirit), and our old self and our old mind (guided by the flesh) are existing side by side. That is why what we don't want to do we still do, like eat that second or third piece of pie. Likewise, what we want to do, like pray and read our Bible for one hour every morning, we just can't seem to make a regular part of our lives. This part of my mind says to do the better thing, but I abruptly do the wrong thing. You may think it is some kind of brain malfunction.

Preacher and evangelist D. L. Moody even confessed, "I have had more trouble with myself than with any other man I have ever met!"[111] The truth is, many believers have a hard time throwing off old habits and self-talk—fleshing out the flesh—and relying totally on God.

Most of us struggle with one form or another of stress, control, anger, submission, money, fear, self-pity, perfection, approval from one another, overeating, or work. We say, "Do you think I really want to do this? I know it's stupid, but it's no use. I yam what I yam. I try to change, but I can't!" Often, someone will use the old nature as an excuse to not change. Self-pity is a roadblock to maturity, plus it keeps other people at bay!

Conquering toxic thoughts and emotions is to acknowledge our pre-Christian experience—the flesh (Romans 7). I take ownership for my feelings and actions. Flesh is my physical body, my habits and memories. It is the inclination of my physical body to fall to the temptation of sin. I am normal (well, pretty much, I think).

Let's break this down. In Christ, I have been set free from the dominion and power of sin (Rom. 6:14), but I still experience life on earth with a physical body and nature to sin. My body is not intrinsically bad, but can be used for evil purposes: I gossip. I watch ungodly programming. I eat too much. I eavesdrop.

When Paul wrote, "We died to sin; how can we live in it any longer?" (Rom. 6:2), he was not referring to the act of committing sins, but to continuing to live under the authority of sin. We must differentiate between the *activity* of sin, which every

Kimberly Davidson

believer lives with, and the *dominion* of sin, which defines the unbeliever.

"While the *presence* of sin can never be abolished in this life, nor the *influence* of sin altered (its tendency is always the same), its *dominion* can, indeed, must be destroyed if a man is to be a Christian" (Sinclair Ferguson).[112]

How do we battle our flesh? Daily, we submit ourselves completely to God. This is will-driven behavior which comes from a healthy brain, versus brain-driven behavior. *Will-driven* behavior is goal directed and productive.[113]

For example, I attended seminary. I often considered it a tribulation because I don't consider myself a natural student. With God as my strength, I embraced this role of student and worked diligently over a period of five years to graduate, despite the many obstacles the enemy and my flesh put in the way.

Brain-driven behavior occurs when the brain hijacks your will, causing you to act in ways that are unhelpful or even downright destructive.[114] My role as a Christian leader is led by the Spirit (most of the time)—will-driven, as in your will be done, Lord! But my role as a woman who can be compulsively concerned with her appearance is led by the flesh—brain-driven. The old me spent a lot of money on cosmetic and facial treatments (brain-driven). The new me knows this is a foolish waste of God's money (will-driven).

When the old me feels pressure by the culture to take action to (attempt) look younger, my flesh begins to fight my Spirit so I R.E.S.I.S.T. First, I pull up Scripture (and tell myself aging is important only if you're cheese or wine!). 1 Corinthians 6:12: "Everything is permissible for me—but not everything is beneficial. Everything is permissible for me, but I will not be mastered by anything."

Second, rather than trying to kill her off, I embrace her and compromise. Instead of expensive treatments, the new me purchases from a selection of reasonably priced products. The flesh gets something, and the Spirit is okay because it's not a sin ... as long as I don't allow my appearance and cosmetic products to become an idol. There's nothing wrong with caring for the outer appearance. But as moms and mentors we should model self-controlled lifestyles. Never forget that any good thing can become an idol if carried to excess.

Why bring up the concept of will-driven versus brain-driven? None of us have the same level of free will. Not one person is the same. All you have to do is look at certain families and observe how very different each child is even though they were created from the same parents. Free will varies on a scale of zero to one hundred. A person with a healthy brain has nearly 100 percent free will. People with OCD or drug addiction or Alzheimer's or ADD are examples of people with virtually no free will. Even a brain scan of a murderer compared to a convicted felon is often dramatic.[115]

Reflect: When you find your flesh in a tug of war with your spirit answer these questions:

1. Is this beneficial and constructive? Will it promote my spiritual life?

2. Is this a practice that over time will tend to master me or become an idol?

3. Will I be a spiritual or fleshly example to others in my life if I do this?

Flesh-Driven versus Holy Spirit-Driven

What we think about and which path we walk is a choice we make each day. Biologically we may not be able to control how much free will we have, but we have been given heavenly power. That gives us hope.

Only God knows just how much of our old mindset will remain. Wherever we are on the free will scale, most of us have enough free will to move forward because of the indwelling presence of the Holy Spirit. "You, however, are controlled not by the sinful nature but by the Spirit, if the Spirit of God lives in you" (Rom. 8:9).

Paul recognized the necessity to yield his life to Christ daily. Paul didn't get stuck like many of us have. He chose to submit to righteous living. As we take action and separate ourselves from the old fleshly thoughts and from toxic products that contaminate our body, we find we want to give up the pleasures of the world and even some old acquaintances.

Carlene desired to break the mindhold of perfection in her life. Perfection to Carlene meant continually cultivating the perfect body and home. She was a chronic dieter and each year spent thousands of dollars redecorating and renovating her home.

For the past year, she consciously worked to replace negative thoughts about her body and perfectionism with positive ones. She quit pointing out every flaw in her and her home. She memorized Scripture and read several Christian self-help books. But day after day, perfectionist Carlene kept resurfacing. Her thinking hadn't changed much.

I suggested she set aside at least thirty minutes a day for God. Through prayer, reading his word, and honest submission, she began seeking the source of her perfectionism. *Reveal the why Lord!* For the first time, she was in a relationship with God. Today she laughs at herself regularly.

Carlene recalled several childhood conversations with Mom. Mom was a perfectionist and ever so conscious about keeping a trim figure. Every mom wants her daughter to feel confident in her own skin, but many often unconsciously impose their own body image blueprint: *You'd be so pretty if...* Her next step was to allow the Holy Spirit time to begin breaking these mindholds from her past. She also chose to meet with a Christian counselor to examine her relationship with her mom.

Our thoughts are extraordinarily powerful. So powerful that when distorted and led by our flesh, they rob us of joy. Every thought we have sends electrical signals though our brain. They have significant influence over every cell in your body. When your mind is burdened with many negative thoughts, it affects the deep limbic system and causes problems such as irritability, moodiness, depression, etc.[116]

The other part of the equation is the body affects the spirit. Jesus told the disciples, "The spirit is willing, but the body is weak" (Matt. 26:41). Often our spirit is motivated to follow God's will but our body is tired or stressed in some way. Then we are not able to do what we should do, like pray or encourage someone. God understands this.

Reflect: The good news is any toxic thought or emotion or attitude is controllable, which means your spiritual, emotional, and physical well-being are controllable too.

If I have confessed and repented of the things I feel guilty or unChristlike about, and I still feel guilty and unChristlike, I recognize this condemnation comes from the enemy, not Jesus. "You cannot tailor-make the situations in life, but you can tailor-make the attitudes to fit those situations" (Zig Ziglar).[117]

People Challenges

As a parent, we often demand that our kids hang out with the "right" group of kids. We know they will mimic another's behavior in order to feel accepted. You are who you spend time with. We too might face people in our lives who either consciously or unconsciously, attempt to sabotage us. They pull us back into the old role or old habits. Who you spend time with matters. When you spend time with pessimistic or hostile people, you tend to feel tense, anxious, sick and not alert. There is classic saying, "If you want to soar with the eagles, don't hang out with turkeys."

If you live with a person that constantly belittles you, you will need to flee. Find others who build you up. No one wields more influence over you than your family and friends. The Scriptures advise, "The righteous should choose his friends carefully. He who walks with the wise grows wise, but a companion of fools suffers harm" (Prov. 12:26; 13:20). Satan wants nothing more than to see us go back down the old, destructive path, living from our flesh, brain-driven, and influenced solely by the world.

There are times you are powerless to remove ungodly influences. You can still remove yourself from the temptation. Let's say you live at home. Your family watches violent movies, drinks a lot, and fights all the time. Until now, you have followed in their footsteps, but now you want to break free. You recognize you need to flee, but you are financially dependent on your family.

You have figured out if you can stay away until they go to bed, you don't get trapped. What are your options in the evening? Go over to a friend's home or the library. Are there any community and church activities you could get involved with? Can you find a restaurant that will allow you to hang out and read or write in your journal? Be alert to the devil, who will try to shut down your options. Brainstorm options with someone else, like your pastor or a mentor or friend.

Reflect: Begin to evaluate your relationships. A healthy relationship includes a balance between giving and taking and honesty with no hint of manipulation. Determine whether they are draining or life-giving.

1. Are you surrounded by people who believe in you and encourage you to do your best and feel good about yourself?

2. Or, do you find yourself in the company of people downplaying or laughing at your ideas?

3. Who are the five people you spend most of your time with? Are they positive or negative?

The Joy Center

Today the pleasure center in the brain is abused, over-stimulated, or taxed beyond its capacities. The result: we can't find real joy in much. We can't even experience the joy that comes from God, which only perpetuates toxic thinking.

Dr. Archibald Hart states that our pursuit of pleasure has skyrocketed. "Today we are relentlessly pushing the pleasure button in our brains and overloading a system that is not designed to be continuously stimulated. The result is *anhedonia*, a condition in which our brain slowly loses the capacity to give us real pleasure."[118]

There is a "joy center" in our brain (it is a scientific term). It is the only area of the brain that grows throughout the life cycle. Every other area of our brain has peak periods and then starts to decline. The joy center is responsible for joy (emotions), rest, and balance. If anyone had cause for being negative, it was Jesus. His life couldn't have been easy, facing satanic opposition and human ridicule. I believe Jesus assessed his joy center. He felt joy because he knew his sufferings could not compare with the joy that awaited him. When we optimize our joy center, we thrive. Our relationships thrive, and we live from the new heart Jesus gave us.[119]

The joy center operates our three basic drives: food, sex, and sleep. The brain regulates each of these basic drives, controlling them automatically and unconsciously. At the same time, our conscious choices and unconscious psychological desires play important roles in how we express these needs. It is no wonder then, when we are upset or wounded, we go to either food, sex, or sleep for comfort.

There are ways to stimulate part of the brain that actually clears the emotional distress generated by the limbic system and also triggers a feeling of well-being. As I have studied the Bible over the years, I too have discovered that knowledge and application of Bible principles and promises have the same effect. God's Word is our daily stress-relieving vitamin.

A woman going through chemotherapy woke up one morning, looked in the mirror, and noticed she had only three hairs left on her head. She thought *I'll braid my hair today*. So she did. She had a wonderful day.

The next day she woke up, looked in the mirror, and had only two hairs on her head. *Hmm*, she thought. *I'll wear a double ponytail today*. She had a grand day.

The following day she woke up and noticed only one hair left on her head. She thought, *What can I do with one hair? A ponytail!* She had a super fun day.

The next day she woke up and noticed there wasn't a single hair on her head. "Yay!" she exclaimed. "I don't have to fix my hair today!" She threw on a beret and had a fabulous day.

She chose to think positive thoughts. She assessed the joy center in her brain. A saying goes: "A thought reaps an action. Action reaps a habit. A habit reaps our character. Our character reaps our destiny."

Reflect: What does the Lord want you to do with this newly acquired knowledge of yourself? Don't let your weaknesses interfere with what you can do. Work to amplify your God-given strengths. There are no shortcuts. A strong mind and foundation only come through work and compliance to what God asks.

A Fruitful Garden

A pastor, in his sermon, told a story about his garden. "I have a garden. In that garden I have the mind of nature. For instance, I know what soil and what seed should produce this, that, and all the other kinds of flowers and fruit. But mark you, the flowers and the fruit are only produced by labor and obedience to the laws of nature. When the garden is beautiful and fruitful, it is only by intelligent cooperation with nature."

Similarly, we Christians have the mind of Christ. Because we are Holy Spirit-driven, we desire to replace negative influences with the fruit of the Spirit: "love, joy, peace, patience, kindness, goodness, faithfulness, gentleness and self-control (Gal. 5:22).

Some of us focus on putting off sinful practices but give little attention to what we put on. Our desire must be to put on the fruit of the Spirit. It is one thing to agree that we need to develop a particular fruit. It is quite another to display that fruit sincerely.

Every Christmas our church becomes part of Prison Fellowship's *Angel Tree,* a ministry that buys gifts for children of prisoners. A few women coordinate it. Since I volunteer for Prison Fellowship, I know how important the *Angel Tree* ministry is to these families. When it comes time for these women to announce the *Angel Tree* ministry, Satan shoots that thought dart: *They should be asking you to join them so you can bear out how important this ministry is. You should really be the one affirming this project!*

My feelings turn into resentment, *I know these prison moms. The church needs my witness!* My attitude changes because I'm feeling rejected. *I just won't talk to them any more!* This is pure self-absorption. Can't you feel the toxicity oozing out? Score: Satan!

The good news is, as a child of God, the fruit of the Spirit is already developing in me. Look at what happens when I choose to step into my role as God's daughter and take a bite of the fruit of the Spirit.

Satan shoots that thought dart: *They should be asking you…*

1. I recognize this is enemy contraband! This dart is coated in pride.

2. Instead of a knee-jerk negative reaction, I pause for sixty seconds and ask the Holy Spirit to help me work through this.

3. I submit and confess my pride. Then I ask for self-control, peace, and love.

4. I interrogate the thought. "I'm feeling this way because I'm jealous, insecure, and controlling. This kind of thinking feeds my flesh. Therefore, I'm not going to react maliciously."

5. I choose to feed the Spirit and replace my thought with, "This is their ministry, their time to be up front, and not mine."

6. My emotions calm back down. My mind is reprogrammed. My attitude changes to "I want to be as supportive as I can."

7. I repent. I ask them what I can do to help.

Kimberly Davidson

8. I thank the Lord for the fruit of the Spirit. I cannot control my circumstances, but I can control my thoughts and emotions ... with God's help.

9. I praise the Lord for what he is doing through these women and *Angel Tree.*

Growing the fruit is the Spirit's doing, unlike indulging the flesh, which is human work. But like a garden that produces luscious and juicy fruit, our spiritual fruit must, too, be tended to, watered, and cultivated. The fruits of the Spirit are only made evident in our lives as we wholeheartedly cooperate with the Lord in full submission and obedience to him by letting his spirit have full control of us—body, soul, and spirit.

Self-control and patience would be an example of a fruit that has to do with our internal thought life, while love and kindness involves external action. Patience is an important Christian virtue. Satan's goal is to instill impatience, get us to give up, as he tried with Job. Like us, Job did become impatient and did not understand what God was doing. But he knew he could trust God.

Faith and patience go together. The flesh is always impatient and leads to costly mistakes. Abraham became impatient waiting for his promised son and "married" Hagar, his wife's maidservant. The son who was born caused nothing but trouble. Satan knows if he can push our impatient button, he can lead us to do something stupid. As they say, idle your motor and put on patience, even when you really feel like stripping the gears!

This list may seem intimidating, and certainly working all nine of these traits into our lives seems impossible, which it is! Our flesh will use any opportunity to indulge itself—if we allow it to. Success only becomes possible when we become dependant on the Holy Spirit to begin producing Christ's character in us. The Spirit teaches us self-control so we will have strength to obey and do what is right in the face of a TAD (temptation, accusation and deception).

Dr. Jerry Bridges, author of *Respectable Sins,* calls this *dependent responsibility.*

We are responsible before God to obey His Word, put to death the sins of our lives, both the so-called acceptable sins and the obviously not acceptable ones. At the same time, we do not have the ability within ourselves to carry out this responsibility. We are in fact totally dependent upon the enabling power of the Holy Spirit. In this sense, we are both responsible and dependent.[120]

How quickly you will bear fruit depends upon how completely you submit yourself to the Holy Spirit's activity. Whether or not your natural temperament or personality is inclined toward or is averted from disciplined thinking, the presence of the Holy Spirit equips you with enough of the supernatural spirit called self-discipline enabling you to sow to the Spirit and not to your flesh. We reap good decisions when we submit to the Spirit.

This doesn't mean we will never see traces of immoral desires again. We no longer live under the authority or power of sin. As we grow in Christ, we are freed from the influence of our self-centeredness, the evil, and the surrounding world. Everything we do flows from a heart of gold and the Spirit. We don't have to sin.

Reflect: Reject the idea there's not much you can do about sin except keep your confessional up to date. In what ways or what areas can you now say your heart and mind are renewed?

The Shack

As the Spirit rebuilds more and more of the person into the new life, the struggles of the old life are reduced. Amen! The aim of sanctification, an act of the Spirit, is to be transformed into the image of Christ.[121] As this happens, the domain of the flesh shrinks. The battle between the old personality role is still there, but her territory is smaller. The spiritual woman is winning! The other awesome thing that happens is as our behavior changes, our brain chemistry changes for the better.

Kimberly Davidson

The assurance that God no longer holds my sin against me frees me. It assures me that God is for me. I am not alone in this battle against Satan, my flesh, and the world. God doesn't wait for me to get my act together. Rather he comes alongside of me.

When we moved to Oregon, we bought a beautiful piece of property on a river with basically a shack on it. But, the shack had a decent foundation. Because the building restrictions were more lenient if we remodeled, that is what we decided to do. In our county, *remodel* meant keeping the foundation and two existing walls. The builders reinforced the foundation. They made the old walls stronger and then framed in a brand new second floor. The whole process took much longer than we anticipated.

When our home was completed, it looked, smelt, and felt brand new. There's nothing like brand new paint, carpeting, cabinetry, and tile. But quickly we began to notice a number of flaws ... big flaws ... little flaws. At first they really bothered me. I got angry and thought we should sue the contractor! But with time they became less noticeable. Today I see them as a part of the character of the house.

You and I start like that shack. Our old nature, the old mindset, doesn't completely get demolished. In fact, we can't bulldoze our foundation because it contains our soul. Our foundation gets supernaturally stronger with the infusing of the Holy Spirit.

Isaiah proclaimed, "Enlarge your house; build on additions; spread out your home! (Isa. 54:2, TLB) We must enlarge our shack because God's presence will add a new dimension to our minds and ultimately, our lives, family, and church. "Adding on" Christ doesn't mean business as usual. Everything changes. We should expect to have a spirit of optimism.

The Holy Spirit either breaks down or gradually reinforces our old walls until they stand strong on their own. Over time God gives us a new nature when we begin the process of replacing our distorted thinking and behavior with God's truth.

How can you tell what kind of foundation you have? Watch to see what happens when you are hit with a fiery dart or a storm comes blowing in. A mind and life built upon the Word of God will withstand the attacks and storms. As we apply these truths in our lives, we will feel better about who we are and why we do what we do.

Reflect: Mediate on this verse and then describe your shack. Jesus said, "The one who hears my words and does not put them into practice is like a man who built a house on the ground without a foundation. The moment the torrent struck that house, it collapsed and its destruction was complete" (Luke 6:49).

R.E.S.I.S.T. Recap

Recognize that your new mind and your old mind are living side by side, explaining why what you don't want to do, you do. Any toxic thought or emotion or attitude is controllable, which means your spiritual, emotional, and physical well-being are controllable too.

Embrace and evaluate your relationships. Determine whether they are draining or life giving. A healthy relationship includes a balance between giving and taking and honesty with no hint of manipulation.

Submit to God the daily battle with your flesh. Rely on the fruit of the Spirit instead of your flesh when you are put in a compromising situation. The fruits are only made evident as you give the Holy Spirit full control of your body, soul, and spirit.

Identify & Interrogate—Assess the joy center in your brain. You are responsible before God to obey his Word while being totally dependent upon the enabling power of the Holy Spirit to put to death the sins of your life—the acceptable sins and the not acceptable ones.

Set your mind and heart on God. If you have confessed and repented of the old mindset and still feel guilty or unChristlike, most likely you are not setting your eyes on Jesus, thereby allowing condemnation from the enemy to filter through.

Thank and Praise God for the new nature he is refining, renovating, and remolding. Thank him for a beautiful mind that has the ability to make healthy choices.

Turn Your Brain Back On

One woman said that her husband and she would go to a nice restaurant twice a week for good food and companionship. She went on Tuesdays. He went on Fridays. Has anyone ever told you "You better change your thinking"?

It's not easy because we're talking about something deeper than thinking. We're talking about convictions held in both our mind and heart. Having been a captive of an eating disorder for seventeen years, I can tell you firsthand how very easy it is to hang onto our mindholds, especially in times of stress.

Scientific data validates we can heal the deep limbic system and change our brain. It requires healing moment-to-moment thought patterns.[122] Automatic toxic thinking (ATT) all has to do with brain chemistry and competence. There are four stages of competence (our capability of performing functions).

One—Unconscious incompetence: I mess up without realizing it. I don't know why I messed up, perhaps generational thinking. Before our new birth, our hearts were hardened and dark. Unknowingly, all we do is sin. Our brain is programmed at stage one.

Two—Conscious incompetence: I am discontented but aware something needs improving. This is the beginning of denying myself. I begin to reject indulging myself according to the world's rules because I aim to please God. My brain is being reprogrammed to stage two.

Three—Conscious competence: I thoughtfully choose to act morally and good. I take action and separate myself from the old fleshly thoughts, toxic foods, and harmful products. My brain is becoming reprogrammed to stage three.

Four—Unconscious competence: I automatically know what is right and wrong and act accordingly. With the Holy Spirit living within me, I am now able to make good decisions. I chose to "put on" love, which binds us all together in perfect unity (Col. 3:12–14). My brain is reprogrammed to stage four.

At stage four, we are able to follow God's commands: we clothe ourselves with compassion, kindness, humility, gentleness, and patience. We bear with each other and forgive whatever grievances we may have against one another.

Reflect: What stage are you at today? Explain your progress, or try to explain what is hindering your from moving to the next stage.

The Limbic Connection

Our overall state of mind is largely based on the types of thoughts we think. When the deep limbic system of the brain is overactive, it sets the mind's filter on "negative." Limbic stress is the greatest enemy of quality of life because it drains the joy out of life. Without the ability to clear or change it, we are only able to function at a small fraction of our potential.

The limbic system doesn't have a memory and doesn't know the difference between yesterday and thirty years ago, explaining why some of our childhood traumas are so powerful today. The limbic system can be negatively programmed through traumatic experiences such as abuse, or the use of drugs and alcohol, or any other compulsive behaviors. These are programmed into the limbic system to avoid uncomfortable thoughts and feelings. They are a substitute for making healthy responses to resolve fear.[123]

For example, Tara's limbic system learned that having needs in a dysfunctional family resulted in vulnerability, hurt, abandonment, and isolation. Now she has to find a new way of thinking—a survival mechanism. One way she does this is by thinking (believing the lie), *I don't need anybody. If I don't need anybody, I'm not vulnerable. If I'm not vulnerable, I don't get hurt.*

Kimberly Davidson

Every time a feeling of vulnerability is experienced, fear says, "Warning!" She flees from a potential blow to the heart.

When the lens we look through is gray or distorted, we are suffering from ATT. Scientific evidence confirms the key to naturally creating inner peace and joy is available without using alcohol or drugs or overeating. The PBS series, *The Brain,* states there are more possible pathways in the brain than there are atoms in the entire known universe. The enhanced joy and improved performance possible with such an unlimited network is incalculable![124]

Our thoughts are worth identifying and interrogating. They can either help or hurt your brain. When a toxic thought slips through the sieve, your mind believes it, and your body reacts to it. Left unchecked, the ATTs will contaminate your whole body system.

Whenever you notice an ATT, pull it down. Take it captive. It's out of commission because it's been killed by the blood of Jesus. It can't affect you anymore. As a child of God, we are given part of Christ's mind (1 Cor. 2:12–16). He has given himself to you and now makes your mind his home.

Reflect: Do you see a familiar ATT in the following list? Yes—counter it with the truth. You can also use the subject index or concordance in the back of your Bible to find the precise verses that speak to your specific situation.

You say: "It's impossible"
God says: All things are possible
(Luke 18:27)

You say: "I'm too tired"
God says: I will give you rest
(Matt.11:28-30)

You say: "Nobody really loves me"
God says: I love you
(John 3:16 & John 3:34)

You say: "I can't go on"
God says: My grace is sufficient
(2 Corinthians 12:9 & Psalm 91:15)

You say: "I'm not smart enough"
God says: I give you wisdom
(1 Corinthians 1:30)

You say: "I can't do it"
God says: You can do it through me
(Philippians 4:13)

You say: "I'm not able"
God says: I am able
(2 Corinthians 9:8)

You say: "It's not worth it"
God says: It will be worth it
(Roman 8:2)

You say: "I can't forgive myself"
God says: I forgive you
(I John 1:9 & Romans 8:1)

You say: "I can't manage"
God says: I will supply all your needs
(Philippians 4:19)

You say: "I'm afraid"
God says: I havn't given you a spirit of fear
(2 Timothy 1:7)

You say: "I'm always worried, frustrated"
God says: Cast all your cares on *me*
(I Peter 5:7)

You say: "I don't have enough faith"
God says: I've given you a measure of faith
(Romans 12:3)

You say: "I feel all alone"
God says: I will never leave you
(Hebrews 13:5)

Limbic Lag

Mind renewal requires exposing the deception, false beliefs, traumatic memories and replacing them with grace, truth, and love. God needs time, and he designed our brain in the same fashion. This is the key to understanding why it takes time. There is a time lag between what your brain *believes* (the limbic system) and what your brain has *learned* (the neocortex). This is called *limbic lag*, a process that can take anywhere from a couple of months to years. The good news is it gets shorter as you continue to challenge and keep taking captive TADs and ATTs.[125]

ATTs tend to rear their ugly heads when we're tired or stressed. This is exactly what Satan wants—to revel in bondage to our own negative thoughts. He wants us totally immersed and consumed in our problems, bound to him by our hurts, fears, and pain. Then we see everything from our own horizontal viewpoint and not from God's perspective. Proverbs 14:12 says, "There is a way that seems right to a man, but in the end it leads to death."

No mind change, no life change! What is learned can be unlearned. What you have believed can be unbelieved when replaced by the truth. Don't get frustrated with God's timetable. Trust him. There is a reason your ATTs aren't changed quickly or easiThink of your mind like a large, clear vase filled with dirty, murky water. Your job is to fill the vase with clear, fresh water until it is no longer dirty and cloudy. The clincher is—you only have an eyedropper to do it. After adding the first few drops, you don't see any change. This is when you may be tempted to give up. That's the devil.

We keep running our thoughts through our brain's filter system. Eventually the water is less dingy. The more drops of water you add, and the more lies that are replaced by truth, the cleaner the water, your mind, becomes. While there will be residual effects, you have made significant improvements. Believe it!

The Bible describes this clean water theory, "Whatever

is true, whatever is noble, whatever is right, whatever is pure, whatever is lovely, whatever is admirable—if anything is excellent or praiseworthy, *think about such things*. Whatever you have learned or received or heard from me, or seen in me—*put it into practice. And the God of peace will be with you*" (Phil. 4:8–9, *my emphasis*). Do not believe every first thought that pops in. Paul is saying that if a thought is not true, don't let it enter your mind!

This is too hard! No it's not. Think back to when you bought a new car. After purchasing the car, you notice the same car everywhere. Suddenly there are hundreds. Before you purchased the car, there were none. They were always there, you simply didn't notice them before. Because you put thought and effort into selecting this particular car, your mind notices this type of car wherever you go.

The same thing happens when you identify negative thinking. You recognize the ATTs everywhere you go, and you become empowered to toss them out. So smile at the woman that just snubbed you. In fact, go one step further and encourage her. Note how good you feel after you have encouraged someone else.

Reflect:

1. Begin to list and identify each ATT that needs to be removed.

2. Replace them with God's thoughts (Scripture).

3. Interrogate: Where did those thoughts originate? This requires prayer and time.

4. Write out the event associated with each ATT. Those ATTs just lost their power.

5. Begin to train yourself to recognize the ATTs. Then write them down and talk to God about them straight from your heart.

The State of Your Brain

In the comic strip *Peanuts*, Linus said, "I love mankind; it's people I can't stand." People can be rude, obnoxious, selfish, foolish and vicious. Some of them are even our enemies—people who criticize us, take advantage of us, or even try to destroy us. We naturally feel resentment, anger, fear, and even hatred.

For some people these suggestions may not work. Certain brain systems are involved in specific behaviors and cause identifiable problems when they "misfire." My husband has a friend who is the very definition of a pessimist and is stubborn headed. Many of the decisions he makes, to me, are crazy. He's also a Viet Nam vet. I am now convinced that being a soldier in that war, combined with a number of helicopter crashes, has affected his entire personality in a depressive way.

I asked myself, "What does Dan's brain look like? Does he say those things and make those nutty decisions because he enjoys irritating other people with his stubbornness? Or, is his brain misfiring because of what happened to him in the past?" I don't know the answer to that. It makes sense to me that his brain is abnormal. I choose to believe that because then I feel sympathy, instead of bitterness, towards him.

According to the National Institute of Mental Health (NIMH), 49 percent of the U.S. population at some point in their lives will suffer from a brain illness, most commonly, anxiety, depression or substance abuse.[126]

Dr. Amen tells the story of a couple in marriage counseling for three years. According to the wife, the husband had changed for the worst over the past several years. Counseling failed. The therapist advised them to divorce $25,000 later. Dr. Amen scanned the husband's brain. His brain showed toxic damage similar to a drug abuser. He denied using drugs. The doctor learned he worked in a furniture factory. The fumes had caused his brain to malfunction—to misfire. He was treated and his marriage saved! And his wife, instead of labeling her husband a jerk, now felt compassion towards him because it was an environmental condition that caused his toxic behavior.

Had this man not looked to the medical-science community their lives would have forever changed for the worst.[127] This is not to say the devil wasn't firing fiery toxic darts into their minds during the counseling process. It makes you wonder how many relationships suffer because one person has a brain problem that no one is aware of.

Some things we might trace back to giving the devil a foothold, but not all of them. With a good brain you will have better relationships, more love in your life, and do good for more people.[128] That's joy and freedom.

Reflect and laugh: A (self-centered) man was walking along a California beach deep in prayer, "Lord, please answer my prayer. Would you build a bridge to Hawaii so I can drive over anytime?"

The sky clouded and a booming voice said, "Your request is very materialistic. Take some time to think of another wish, a wish you think would honor and glorify me."

The man thought for a long time and finally said, "Lord, I wish I could understand women's minds. I want to know what they feel inside, what they are thinking when they give me the silent treatment, why they cry, what they mean when they say *nothing* and *I'm fine!*. And how I can make a woman truly happy?"

There was dead, darkening silence. A few moments later God said, "How many lanes do you want on that bridge?"

You Think What You Eat

The Genesis of Our Down Fall by Jordan Rubin[129]

In the beginning God created the heavens and the earth, and He populated the earth with vegetables, fruits of all kinds, seeds and grains and healthy animals to provide meat and dairy products, all so Man and Woman could live long and healthy lives. Then Satan created ice cream and glazed donuts. And Satan said to Man, "You want chocolate with that?" And Man replied, "Yes!" and Woman said, "As long as you're at it, add some sprinkles. Man and Woman gained ten pounds and Satan smiled...

God then gave grass-fed beef rich in iron and zinc and low in fat so that Man and Woman might consume more minerals and fewer calories. But Satan created fast-food restaurants and 99-cent double cheese burgers. Then he said, "You want fries with that?" "Yes! And supersize them! Man replied. Satan said, "It is good," and Man went into cardiac arrest. God sighed and created quadruple bypass surgery.

Food is the bait Satan uses to tempt us, over and over again, until it finally becomes a mindhold, often with deadly consequences. Ironically, our culture bombards us with ads that promote illness! Even Solomon pointed out, "All man's efforts are for his mouth, yet his appetite is never satisfied" (Eccl. 6:7). What does your diet consist of?

1. Raw fruits and vegetable, hearty wheat bread and granola.
2. Chocolate cheesecake, ice cream, and Alka Seltzer.
3. Anything that can be bought at the golden arches.

Bill Cosby said, "I am what I ate...and I'm frightened." Therapists say eating is one of our earliest nurturing memories, explaining why many of us try to comfort ourselves with food. More women struggle with food and diet than anything else.

Researchers have discovered a long-held truth: foods generate a profound effect in the human brain. Literally, you think what you eat. Food is as powerful as any medicine that science can design.130 When we eat right, we feel better, sleep better, and have a sunnier disposition. Eat wrong, like starting with a couple of donuts, and you feel lethargic, stupid, and cranky—

very unChristlike. Our thoughts can careen out of control if our diet is not balanced. That certainly explains some people's behavior, doesn't it?

Our diet is often our identity. Tina loves to cook for her family, but she barely eats. She is determined to stay thin. Thin this week is ninety-five pounds. She restricts her daily diet to seven hundred calories. Daily her small frame weakens, yet she thinks, *If I lose a few more pounds, then I'll be truly happy.* This is an example of inadequate nutrition impairing the brain.

Reflect: Keeping our mind and body healthy is work. It's important everyday to eat a balanced diet, exercise properly, and focus on the right target—God. Paul said, "Put on the Lord Jesus Christ, and make no provision for the flesh in regard to its lusts" (Rom. 13:14, NASB). In other words, get rid of it. What we don't have in the pantry, we're far less likely to have on our hips!

Mind Nutrition

No one said this was going to be easy. In fact Paul, himself, said, "Like an athlete I punish my body, treating it roughly, *training it to do what it should,* not what it wants to" (1 Cor. 9:27, TLB, *my emphasis*). You can do this! Keep going!

Thought nutrition consists of ingesting protein foods for mental performance; carbohydrates serve as the brain's main energy source. We actually need to eat fat—good fats that contain omega 3 and 6 that we get from fish, eggs, nuts and seeds. Vitamin D, "the sunshine vitamin," is important to brain health. A deficiency may contribute to brain-related diseases. When you eat, sit down and eat slowly. Your brain needs twenty minutes to register that you are full.

Water (God's nectar) is the nutrient transportation system to the brain. We need to drink lots of it, a good six glasses a day, for optimum function of all body systems. Water is the most important non-food for your body. It aids in fat metabolism, helps concentration, alertness and muscle tone. It improves mood, regulates blood pressure, detoxifies and decreases water retention.[131]

Hormone Hostages

Every hormone hostage knows there are days in the month when all a man has to do is open his mouth and he takes his life in his hands. What does PMS actually stand for? "Pass My Shotgun, Psychotic Mood Disorder, Perpetual Munching Spree, Puffy Mid Section, Pardon My Sobbing," and my favorite, "Pass My Sweatpants."

Premenstrual syndrome is real. During PMS, our brain chemistry is genuinely altered and produces reactions we cannot control. The deep limbic system has a higher density of estrogen receptors than other parts of the brain, making it more vulnerable.[132] For the woman who is what some might call crazed— *I'm out of estrogen and have a gun, so leave me alone*—physicians can prescribe appropriate medications.

Exercise

We know fat is bad for our overall health (obesity lops off as much as 20 years of life), but did you know it's bad for your brain? Research from Kaiser Permanente found those with the fattest arms at ages 40 to 45 were 59 percent likely to have dementia later in life. Another study found those with particularly large bellies at midlife, were 260 percent more likely to develop dementia.[133] One solution: exercise. It helps to sharpen thinking by oxygenating the brain and optimizing mental performance. It slows brain shrinkage, builds strength and lowers stress.

The Power of Sleep

Get at least seven to eight hours of sleep per night to support your metabolic rate and allow your muscles and soft tissues to heal from exercise. If you are sleep deprived your metabolic rate will slow down to conserve energy![134]

Our culture minimizes the importance of sleep. *I'm too busy to sleep.* There is a lot of data showing that sleep stabilizes, strengthens, and integrates our memories. It gives our brain a chance to regroup and consolidate information. Lack of sleep also makes you cranky! And have you noticed when we're cranky we're less cute?

Studies on sleep deprivation found people who get less than eight hours of sleep experience pronounced cognitive and physiological deficits. This includes impairment in memory, decision-making, and attention. Researchers also found the language center shuts down in the brains of healthy young people who took a simple word test after staying awake for thirty-five hours.[135] This explains why I have mush-mouth when I'm sleep deprived!

The effects go beyond the brain. Our immune system suffers as well. Metabolism is disrupted, and there is growing evidence for a link between sleeplessness and obesity. I know when I am sleep deprived I crave carbohydrates and tend to overeat. Research has shown that insufficient sleep appears to tip hunger hormones out of whack.

Reflect: You have just completed Part Three: *Refocusing the Present and the Future.* Let's do a self-check exercise to see how you are doing so far.

1. Are you still guilt beating? How many "could of," "would of," "should of" or "if onlys" were part of your vocabulary this week?

2. How many "always" or "never" statements have you uttered today?

3. How many conversations have you replayed in your head recently?

4. How many fortune-telling, "what if this happens in the future" scenarios have you created?

5. How much of your time is spent mind reading or speculating what other people are thinking (even when they haven't told you anything)?

6. Are you focusing only on the negative, seeing the bad in every situation?

7. Are you (or have you) forming an identity around your problem, diet or disease?

8. Do you blame others for your problem? Do you feel like a victim, that everything you touch goes wrong because what has happened to you?

9. Do you think without interrogating your feelings? "I think this, so it must be!"

If you answered yes to even one of these, continue to work on pulling down and interrogating these toxic mindholds. Keep a diary of emotional eating or sleep depravation incidents and develop alternatives, such as journaling, praying, listening to music, and going to bed earlier.

R.E.S.I.S.T. Recap

Recognize all of your actions are the result of the way you think. When an automatic toxic thought (ATT) slips through, your mind believes it and your body reacts to it. Left unchecked, ATTs will contaminate your whole body system.

Embrace each ATT and take it captive. It's out of commission. List all ATTs that need to be removed. Write out the event associated with each ATT. Then replace it with truth (Scripture). What you have believed can be unbelieved.

Submit your burdens to God and turn your thoughts to positive and God-honoring things. God doesn't tell you what not to do, but he gives you the "to think on" list—Philippians 4:8–9.

Identify & Interrogate—Where did those ATT thoughts originate? Begin to train yourself to recognize the ATTs. Then write them down and talk to God about them. What is learned can be unlearned.

Set your mind and heart on God. Do not to believe every first thought that pops into your head. Run it through your brain's filter system. Set your mind on drinking plenty of water and getting adequate exercise and rest. Keep a diary of emotional eating or sleep depravation incidents and develop alternatives.

Thank and Praise God for your unique and incredible body. You might have to give up some things, but God doesn't ask you to give up anything that is good for you—only bad. Praise him for caring so much about you.

Part Four

A Transformed Mind

We're free of it! All of us! Nothing between us and God, our faces shining with the brightness of his face. And so we are transfigured much like the Messiah, our lives gradually becoming brighter and more beautiful as God enters our lives and we become like him.

–Paul, 2 Corinthians 3:17–18, The Message

A man [*woman*] must himself [*herself*] be cleansed, before cleansing others; himself [*herself*] become wise, that he [*she*] may make others wise; become light, and then give light; draw near to God, and so bring others near; be hallowed, then hallow them; be possessed of hands to lead others by the hand, of wisdom to give advice.

–Gregory of Nazianzus[136]

I tell you the truth, unless you change and become like little children, you will never enter the kingdom of heaven. Therefore, whoever humbles himself like this child is the greatest in the kingdom of heaven.

–Jesus, Matthew 18:1–4

The Garbage Man
Always Rings Twice

After Carla worked on putting R.E.S.I.S.T. into place, she cheerfully exclaimed to her sister, "I've changed my mind!" Her sister replied, "That's wonderful. Does this one work any better?"

When I say *I changed my mind* in the context of what we have been learning, I am saying I am thinking and acting more like Jesus Christ. To many, this seems impossible. Dr. Roger Walsh, author of *Essential Spirituality*, wrote:

> The mind has a remarkable quality to mirror and take on the qualities of whatever we attend to. If we listen to an angry person or watch a violent scene our minds start to boil with anger. If we focus on a loving person, our mind tends to fill with love. Once this is recognized, two things quickly become apparent: One, if we could control attention, we could concentrate on specific people and memories to evoke desired qualities such as love and joy. Two, what we put into our minds is just as important as what we put into our mouths. Our mental diet affects our mental health ... Wise attention ... cultivates a healthy mind. What we concentrate on we become, and once we can control attention, we can concentrate on anything we wish.[137]

Renewing our minds is not simply changing our thoughts, but actually putting off our old, negative thoughts while putting on God's thoughts. We can't just say "God, give me humility," and somehow expect him to automatically give us his mind of humility. We must cultivate humility for it doesn't come naturally.

To *renew* means to exchange one thing for another. We're exchanging our thinking for God's. If we're not willing to submit our pride—exchange it for humility, then our lives will remain the same. Each time we recognize self-centered thinking, we toss it out and begin the process of confessing, submitting, and repenting of it. Then we are closer to a Christlike mind.

This won't happen overnight, but as we choose to pray and spend time with God, our thinking will change because God works in us. He supplies the will to obey, to act in humility, and do things that please him. That is one of the paradoxes of the Christian life.

Let's suppose I am channel surfing and a program grabs my attention. I begin to watch it and realize it is about a woman who chooses to stay with an abusive husband. As I watch the first love making scene, my body tenses up. When he hits her repeatedly, I become really uncomfortable. Why? I am in Christ and he is in me. I have two choices: One, watch the program and believe I am strong enough and it won't affect me.

Or will it? Our body reacts to every thought we have. Polygraph and lie detector tests confirm this. The second option is to say, "I don't need to watch this because I share in Jesus's divine nature. Even though my flesh is saying one thing, I, as his image bearer, say no. Sin is not my friend but my enemy.

I'm free from the conflict zones. I could have thought to myself, *I won't watch this. I'll make a great sacrifice for Jesus. I'll suffer.* But I don't. I decide not to watch the program because that is not who I am and I actually desire to say no.

Emma Moody (wife of D.L. Moody) said, "You know what you ought to do, then do it, not halfway, but out and out."[138] This is what mind renewal is all about. It's not about existing as a Christian, feeling deprived. It's about exchanging your thinking and discovering the life God has called you to live. You are fulfilling your purpose while at the same time being who you really are. Secondly, changing your actions helps your brain work more efficiently!

Reflective Exercise: A toxic thought dart hits. Before I act, I ask, "Does this thought fit who I am? Is this thought healthy?

Kimberly Davidson

Does it fit my beliefs, character, morals, and values?" No. Confront the intruders: "You're a wicked thought. Be gone, prideful thinking!" Toss it out! Say, "I choose to think about whatever is true, noble, right, pure, lovely, admirable, excellent, or praiseworthy. I choose to focus on a positive and loving person or memory and any awesome thing God has created. This is who I am."

Fasting From Garbage

Teachers today paint a picture of young students lacing their stories with violence, sex, and savagery. Forty-two percent of first-, second-, and third-grade girls want to be thinner. What a stark testimony to the early age at which children are absorbing the ugly and evil side of life. It's *garbage in, garbage out.*

We know what goes into our minds often comes out in our words and actions. Entertainment is a great example. Most movies today pull our minds into the gutter. It would not be so damaging if the mind was equipped like a garbage disposal. Then you could churn and flush away all the noxious information and be done with it. The mind doesn't work that way. It stores up impressions for a lifetime. The only way to protect the mind is to expose it to the best.

It wasn't that long ago that I made a decision to fast from nonsensical television shows. Instead of eliminating television altogether, I began watching more creation-based programming (*The Learning Channel, National Geographic, Animal Planet,* the *History* and *Discovery Health Channels*). Creation gives dramatic evidence of God's existence, his power, his love, and his care. It's my way of joining the heavens and the skies in glorifying God (Ps. 19:1–6). I always have something to talk to God about, which strengthens our relationship.

When I say "fasting," what or who comes to mind? John the Baptist types? Legalists? Health nuts … or just nuts? What about Jesus? Fasting, I believe, does not always mean the abstinence from food. Fasting is also a voluntary denial of a normal life function for the sake of intense spiritual activity.139

We may need to fast from involvement with certain people, the media, our cell phone, email, or magazines in order to become more absorbed in a time of spiritual and mind renewal. Limit the amount of time spent playing videos games, watching non-sense television, and reading romance novels. Begin to engage in other activities such as talking to a family member, playing or grooming the dog, clean out and organize your closet, learn a new language, exercise. Go for a walk with God, capturing the majesty of his creation.

The next question is: "For how long?" Nowhere in Scripture are we asked to fast for forty days or for any specific length of time. One principle we can learn from Jesus is that fasting is a way of overcoming temptation and beginning anew, dedicating ourselves to God. The Bible says that fasting may be an act of devotion to God (see Luke 2:37).

Reflect: Write down how many times a day you interact with all types of media (TV, computer, cell phone, DVD). Compare that to how many times a day you participate in a faith-based exercise (reading your Bible, or listening to Christian radio, a sermon CD or music). Will you fast as the Holy Spirit directs?

Festering Anger

Not too long ago, my buttons were pushed and festering toxic anger erupted. You could say I lost it. I literally took Jesus's words out of context: "If your brother sins against you, go and show him his fault, just between the two of you" (Matt. 18:15). I did just that because I was convinced my anger was righteous and justified. She needed to hear what I had to say. I saved Jesus the job of having to do it! But afterwards I felt horrible … sick.

Revenge and personal justice didn't feel as good as I thought it would. I felt bad because I sinned. Proverbs 16:32 says "better a man [*woman*] who controls his [*her*] temper." Jesus taught

Kimberly Davidson

that what we say begins in the heart (Luke 6:45). Paul taught love does not envy or boast, is not proud, rude, nor self-seeking (1 Cor. 13:4–5). All these ugly things spring from our flesh, and Satan antagonizes the situation.

In retrospect, I wished I practiced what I preach. When we get angry, it is important to practice putting separation between our emotions and our words. Hit the pause button. I prayed…and prayed more about it. *Help me Jesus!* I felt he instructed me to tell her where this anger came from and ask for her forgiveness (Matt. 5:24). I did that immediately. Naturally, I thought her reaction would be, "I'm so sorry I hurt you. Of course I forgive you!" In her eyes this was another attack—just hidden behind the cross.

The damage is done when our emotions take a shortcut through our brain and head straight to our tongue. Every verse that speaks to keeping our mouths shut and turning the other cheek came to the forefront of my mind, like Proverbs 10:19–20 and Matthew 5:39. I had been hurt, but now I was the one feeling guilty.

Through prayer I began to see the errors of my ways. I confessed and repented, but I couldn't get this incident out of my mind. This entire episode had taken the form of a big, stinky garbage can. I sifted through it and found what was stinking it up: judgment and criticism and stubborn pride.

I clearly saw how my anger played out: as judge and jury. *Kimberly, put your judge's robe into the garbage can. Give it to Jesus.* Biblically, I was wrong. Scripture commands us not to judge or condemn (Luke 6:37). It also tells us God will treat us with the same grace or severity with which we treat others (Luke 6:38).

Help me Jesus! I can't let go of this garbage. What do I do next? It was like he said, "*You* do nothing. Give *me* the garbage. You've done a fabulous job of acknowledging and sifting through it. Now give your garbage to me. I'll dispose of it."

I imagined wheeling this garbage can over to Jesus. He smiled and wheeled it away. Jesus will do a much better job than I as judge. Some time when by…What's that smell, that obnoxious odor? I looked around. The garbage can is back! I kept replaying what happened over and over in my mind and it would make me angry all over again.

By not forgiving, we actually give control of our emotional state to the person we're angry with. It allows them to control our lives through the constant replaying of that mind tape, reinforcing the pain. I began to ask Jesus, "What words and actions could have reversed this toxic situation and turned it into a positive experience? Help me change my mind toward her and to try to see her as you see her."

I didn't have all the information—like the condition of her heart and brain. I know she is not a happy person. She hasn't been content for years. Perhaps her arrogance is her way of blotting out that hurt. I cannot change the past but I can change the future. I trust God to take this situation and work it out according to his plan ... not mine, freeing me. The thief comes only to destroy—to instigate anger and destroy relationships, but Jesus came that we may have life, and have it to the full (John 10:10).

Reflect: "In facing up to our anger, we need to realize that no one else causes us to be angry. Someone else's words or actions may become the occasion of our anger, but the cause lies deep within us—usually our pride, or selfishness, or desire to control" (Dr. Jerry Bridges).[140] Think of the last time you said something you regretted. Interrogate your anger. What is the deep lying cause?

Breaking Mindholds with a Forgiving Spirit

A reporter wrote, "Never before, say some experts, has there been such a need to forgive what seems to be the unforgivable." Turn on the news and you can understand this statement. The solution: send her or him to an anger management class! Do we really want to merely manage our anger? Let's talk about anger resolution.

Often we hold resentment or bitterness in our hearts because we don't identify these emotions as sinful anger. For many of us, anger and bitterness have become our identity. We tend to focus on the other person's offense justifying our own behavior because we don't see it as an offense. Regrettably, sinful anger always leads to more sin, hurting ourselves as well as others.

Many of us are stuck because we are still held captive by mindholds of anger and unforgiveness, instead of being captivated by God's amazing grace and forgiveness. Many women believe they don't deserve forgiveness for themselves. They are very good at forgiving others but are not able to eliminate their own guilt.

Only the power and blood of Jesus can remove the remnants of our own self-inflicted guilt. A nurse once said there are three phrases that matter most in life: "Forgive me," "I forgive you," and "I love you." Love keeps no record of wrongs (1 Cor. 13:5).

Unforgiveness comes in many forms, such as bitterness, broken trust, hatred, humiliation, malice, a shattered self-image, grudges and resentment (James 4:1–3). It can plant a "root of bitterness" ruining the work of the fruit of the Holy Spirit, stunting spiritual growth, and contributing to physical illness. When we hurt our defense mechanism is anger. We hang onto it as a means of protection.

Bitterness is one of the best disguised mindholds. Like acid can destroy the vessel that holds it, unforgiveness can destroy us. It is like drinking poison and hoping the other person gets ill…and they usually don't! Unforgiveness only gives you tense muscles, a headache, wrinkles, and a sore jaw from clenching your teeth. If we think we are winning, most likely we are losing.

What does the Bible say? Plenty. "Get rid of all bitterness, rage and anger, brawling and slander, along with every form of malice" (Eph. 4:31). This is a command. Put away—get rid of—*all* anger. That doesn't mean that we cease to have strong convictions or lose our desire for justice. In my previous illustration, I was angry because I felt she was acting arrogant. Arrogance is a sin which we should not overlook. Because it is a sin, I trust that God will deal with her as he deems fit.

"In your anger do not sin: Do not let the sun go down while you are still angry, and do not give the devil a foothold" (Eph.

4:26–27). The Bible doesn't tell us we shouldn't deny conflict, but it points out it is important to handle anger properly. Nip it in the bud! Anger is normal. Repressed or uncontrolled anger is dangerous. We refuse to allow the sins of others to cause us to sin further.

Phyllis Diller said, "Never go to bed mad. Stay awake and fight."[141] She's right from the standpoint it's important to voice our issues as long as we are fighting fair. If not vented thoughtfully, anger has the potential to kill relationships.

We need to answer the questions "What is (or was) *my* part? What did *I* do wrong?" By the time the sun sets, say what is on your mind and let go of the things you can't change. Carrying the cancer of anger to bed night after night will destroy you.

Granted there is righteous and justified anger, which Jesus expressed. But it is sinful anger that gives the devil a foothold, giving him room to work his nastiness. Satan can exploit, empower, or energize our sin. *Look at how evil he has been to you! He doesn't deserve forgiveness! Never reconcile!*

The Bible tells us we need to deal with our anger immediately in a way that will edify a relationship rather than destroy or divide it. You may not be able to resolve the problem before the sun goes down (by the end of the day), but you can begin to put some step in place and work on it. If you don't, the devil starts construction on a mindhold.

What is *sin* in this verse? It could be related to an unforgiving attitude that accompanies anger or any of the anger emotions. Do not be fooled—a bitter, angry personality can exist inside an otherwise deeply committed Christian. Most of the time it remains hidden until some perceived injustice brings it to the surface. After the explosion, the person returns to her usual Christian equilibrium. But in the cavern of her mind lurks the angry personality, guarding piles of quarrels and grudges.

Do an inventory on the condition of your heart. Anger turned inwards often manifests itself as depression. If you are depressed I suggest pastoral and/or therapeutic counseling. The essence of forgiveness is the surrender of our expectations, rights, and pride to God's will. Turn the other cheek. Grasp repentance and forgiveness. Now you are setting your mind on the things of God and giving him control of your life.

Reflect: Think of the last time you were really mad at someone. You imagine, and you might even have prayed, the worst things happening to this person. If that person were dying, how might that change your attitude now? Explain.

Are you having a problem forgiving someone who has died? Many of us get trapped here. Write that person a letter. Give it to God and allow him to set you free.

Decisional and Emotional Forgiveness

God is very clear on the matter of forgiveness. The devil knows in order for God to forgive us, we must forgive (Mark 11:26). He knows if we choose to withhold forgiveness, our worship and prayers are fruitless (Mark 5:23–24).

The devil may even promote forgiveness. It is not uncommon to rush into expressing forgiveness without processing the underlying pain. The devil will say, *Forgive. It is the right thing to do. Make your family happy!* This is very common in cases of incest. He knows if you forgive without dealing with the underlying causes, he still has you in his dungeon. You will erupt at some point. On the other hand, if the devil can convince you not to forgive someone, which may even be yourself, he wins.

Theodore Roosevelt (the twenty-sixth president) said, "In any moment of decision the best thing you can do is the right thing, the next best thing is the wrong thing, and the worst thing you can do is nothing." There two concepts or types of forgiveness: *decisional* and *emotional.* They don't have to work together, but they usually do.

In the *decisional forgiveness* process I choose to obey God. "Be kind and compassionate to one another, forgiving each other, just as in Christ God forgave you" (Eph. 4:32). I say, "You hurt and wronged me. But I choose not to hold it against you. I trust God to judge you fairly."

It is not a feeling but an act of my will to follow God's Word. I don't want to hold this injustice against you or seek revenge. I want to put this behind me and move on. I am making a decision about my behavioral intentions. My mind is will-driven. And I may have to put some safeguard or boundary into place so this event doesn't happen again.

Shelly wrote her step-father, "You ruined my life—tormented, destroyed, and betrayed me and so I told your dirty little secret even though you said you would hurt or even kill me. God wants me to forgive you, which I do. He'll deal with you."

We will always remember the painful situation or loss, but we choose to take our focus off the offender and set our eyes on God. We say, "Satan, I'm not giving you a foothold in my mind!" Isaiah assures us God supplies perfect peace to those whose thoughts turn often to him (Isa. 26:3). That freedom moves us into the healing phase, back into relationship with God and others.

The second type, *emotional forgiveness,* is the process of replacing negative emotions with positive emotions. With decisional forgiveness I choose to forgive you, but I cannot control my emotions. My mind is brain-driven. I'm still hanging onto the negative emotions of bitterness, anger, hatred, and fear. That stinky garbage can keeps rolling back. We often need the help of a professional counselor or pastor, along with the support of friends. It could also happen quickly depending on the event.

Decisional forgiveness takes place instantaneously, while emotional forgiveness can be a recovery process, taking years to heal depending on how deep the wound. It is the process of emotionally releasing and forgiving, perhaps time and again. And let us also not forget, forgiving and escaping consequences are not synonymous.

Bitterness and anger are weaknesses. Paul taught that God's power is made perfect in our weakness (2 Cor. 12:9). Paul said a further reason for forgiveness is to keep from being outsmarted by Satan, for we know what he is trying to do (2 Cor. 2:11, TLB). God casts our sins into the depths of the sea (Mic. 7:19), and we should do the same with the sins of others. Shelly eventually found emotional forgiveness:

Dad, I found hope. God not only wanted me to survive but to have freedom and joy in my life, which you took away. God is now my Father, and he loves and cares for me. He wants the very best for me—to be whole and healthy again, physically and psychologically. I forgive you. I'm letting you go from the dark recesses of my mind and heart. I let go of the pain, the rage, and the memories. You don't deserve it—I do!

Reflect: The ability to forgive is essential for your spiritual, emotional, and physical well-being:

1. Recognize that until you forgive you are in bondage. Score: Satan!

2. Repent: "Lord, I know I'm not following your commandment to forgive. As you know, I am having difficulty forgiving [name]. However, right now, in your name, through your shed blood, drawing on your strength, I am making a decision to forgive [name]. I take [name] off my hook and place [name] on your hook."

3. "Lord, I thank and praise you for forgiving me and being to so patient and understanding with me ... [talk to God in your own words]."

4. Reaffirm your faith and trust in God by getting right back into his Word.

Putting On A Mind of Love

Helen Keller said, "It is wonderful how much time good people spend fighting the devil. If they would only expend the same amount of energy loving their fellow men, the devil would die in his own tracks."[142] Love is listed as the first fruit of the Spirit.

When you look at your child, do you think with a heart of love or frustration:

1. This child is pure joy!
2. Did I get someone else's baby at the hospital?
3. For this I have cellulite and stretch marks.

"Do not waste time bothering whether you "love" your neighbor; act as if you did. As soon as we do this we find one of the great secrets. When you are behaving as if you loved someone you will presently come to love him… Love is not affectionate feeling, but a steady wish for the other person's ultimate good as far as it can be obtained" (C. S. Lewis).[143]

The Bible tells us, "Be kind and compassionate to one another" (Eph. 4:32). It's certainly easy to love the lovable. What about the angry, irritating people at work or on the freeway or in our church—how are we to love them? Most Christians think that Christian love is a feeling. It is not; it is a decision, a willing, a choice.

In Scripture, all commands of love are verbs not adjectives, like, "Love your enemies" (Matt. 5:44). Do you think Jesus is saying have a warm, affirmative emotion towards them? No. He knows us better. He asks us to do something with our behavior. Love, according to God, is mostly behavior, controlled by our cognitions. It is tied to obedience—to action which involves our will. Jesus said, "If anyone loves me, he will obey my teaching" (John 14:23).

We've got it backwards. Our flesh says, *I will love you when I feel it.* However, we are told by God to "put on love," (Col. 3:14) which means love everybody at all times, even when we don't feel it. Love always needs other verbs to give it hands and feet. Alone it can do nothing.

Paul uses love as a noun. Love is patient, love is kind, it does not envy or boast, and so on (read 1 Corinthians 13: 4–7). We choose to love that person at all times, maybe not in heart, but by our actions. We put on a mind of love. That love gives validity to my actions and makes them acceptable to God. This is obedient love.

Translation: *Do unto others as you would have them do unto you.* I am to love my enemies without regard to my personal feelings towards them. With the Spirit's help, I choose to honor and respect you. However, if I am only kind to my enemies so they will hopefully be nice to me or do something for me, this is not love. It is manipulation. It is my flesh in action, looking out for my welfare under the disguise of looking out for theirs.

It's been said that love is not something you live for. Love is something you become. Love arises in our hearts only as we, by faith, lay hold of the great truths of the Word of God. That is why we must be constantly nourished by feeding on it.

C.S. Lewis affirmed, "The worldly man treats certain people kindly because he "likes" them: the Christian, trying to treat every one kindly, finds himself liking more and more people as he goes on—including people he could not even have imagined himself liking at the beginning."[144]

Reflect: Who is that one person you will, however reluctantly, smile at or hug the next time you see her or him? (Do you have trouble hugging because your family didn't hug? If yes, make a conscious effort to hug one person a day. You can even tell them you are required to hug one person a day. Let God direct you.) Think of a person you can write a love letter to. Both these exercises are extremely powerful.

R.E.S.I.S.T. Recap

Recognize that if you are festering with anger, you may have (or had) a part to play. Answer the questions: "What is/was *my* part? What did *I* do wrong?"

Embrace fasting. Do you need to fast from involvement with certain people, the media, your cell phone, email, or magazines in order to carve out time for spiritual and mind renewal? Are you committed to fast as the Holy Spirit directs?

Submit prideful thinking and exchange it for humility. Submit all your stinky, unforgiving garbage to Jesus. Let him dispose of it. Pray for those who have hurt you.

Identify & Interrogate toxic thoughts by asking: Does this thought fit who I am? Is this thought healthy? Does it fit my beliefs, character, morals, and values? If not, confront and then toss out that thought.

Set your mind and heart on God when you confront any painful memory. Talk to God and at least one other person about it. Then choose to put it off, replacing it with an active memory of God's goodness and faithfulness stored up from your past.

Thank and Praise God that justice and revenge is for him to repay. Make the decision to forgive. Thank him for taking that burdensome heat off you. Praise God that he will walk beside you and enable you eventually to forgive that person emotionally.

A Beautiful Mind

I'll never forget that day when the stick turned blue. *I'm pregnant! Abortion is the only answer.* After all, I had been deceived—it was only a so-called blob of tissue. After the abortion, I chose to bury (repress) this experience like a wrecked ship on the bottom of an ocean. Until I met Jesus. I became keenly aware of the sin I had committed. Once I confessed the abortion, God hit the "clear" button. It was amazing grace!

I accepted God's grace. Coupled with learning the real truth and a group of godly women, I found freedom and joy. With God, we are safe and can reveal our painful secrets. His healing journey encourages us to seek the truth so we can acknowledge the past, the sin, and move forward. Bathed in his grace, we are able to confront and conquer toxic thoughts and emotions.

Grace gives us the privilege of evaluating who we were—our past experiences—against who we are today—image bearers of Jesus. If we continue to revisit the past, and beat ourselves up mentally for either something we did, or for something said to us, the devil is in control. When I give myself grace, I am acknowledging I am forgiven. I give God, the Father, the reigns to control my life.

Grace is God's bountiful supply of our every need. It is the only thing that can bring hope and transformation to this jaded world. We certainly don't deserve it, "When the time came for the kindness and love of God our Savior to appear, then he saved us—not because we were good enough to be saved but because of his kindness and pity—by washing away our sins and giving us the new joy of the indwelling Holy Spirit" (Tit. 3:4–5, TLB). This is grace.

Through his grace God renews our minds and brings us freedom to live a new life. It becomes our motivation to resist temptation and sin, and make righteous choices. "It teaches us to say "No" to ungodliness and worldly passions, and to live self-controlled, upright and godly lives in this present age" (Tit. 2:11–12).

This is the same grace that enabled Jesus to endure the mocking, beatings, and crucifixion at the hands of those whom he came to save. When we have the grace to be free in the presence of those who judge us, we have real Christian freedom.

Reflect: Name two things in your life right now that Satan may be using to keep you from embracing God's grace?

Humility in Our World Today

Isaiah 35:8 tells us that our own natural way of thinking, even as Christians, is not only different than God's, but it's usually totally opposite from God's. Case in point: "Do nothing out of selfish ambition or vain conceit, but in humility consider others better than yourselves. Your attitude should be the same as that of Christ Jesus" (Phil. 2:3, 5).

As we seek God's kingdom on earth and not our own purposes, we gain the same mind as our Father (Matt. 6:10). We become co-laborers with God by praying faithfully and behaving in agreement with his desires. Then we have the capacity to think the way he thinks—if we choose to.

Nobody moves toward a mind of Christ without humility. Most of us are not naturally humble. A famous Christian businessman was speaking at a church. He got carried away boasting to the congregation about all God had given him: a successful business, a large home, a great family, a famous name, and enough money to travel and give to charities. He commented that many people would love to change places with him. Then he exclaimed, "What more could God give me?"

From the back a voice yelled, "A dose of humility!"

Why is it that we eat humble pie when we're forced into an apology or retraction? No one wants to face humiliation for a serious error. Humiliation and humility are not the same, although they often feel the same. "Humility is an eager willingness to see where you are wrong in order to experience the power of God that has already made you fit for His presence" (Dr. Larry Crabb).

Humility is a mysterious trait. Yet, God regards it as a very important characteristic. It means we honestly estimate ourselves, our character, and accomplishments. It is not self-degradation—it's magnifying God. Humility is not stepping down, but standing next to God. When we recognize that our success comes from God, we are then thinking in a humble manner.

Paul wrote to the Romans, "Do not think of yourself more highly than you ought, but rather think of yourself with sober judgment, in accordance with the measure of faith God has given you" (Rom. 12:3). Humility is a state of mind we want to work toward. We replace denial and blame with an attitude of humility and transparency—first, before God so he may begin his refining work in us, then toward others, as a model and encourager.

Jesus proclaimed, "Now that I, your Lord and Teacher, have washed your feet, you also should wash one another's feet" (John 13:14). Jesus did not humble himself in the presence of others because his self-esteem was low. He chose to serve them because of who he was, a God who loves.

If you are ever in doubt about what makes a person great, do not look to the Hollywood elite or the upper crust of society. Importance is not found in possessions, power, or prestige. It is found in service, character, and humility.

Humility requires God-confidence. You know who you are in Christ and choose to serve others. Being able to relieve someone else of some overwhelming tasks or make someone else feel important, without feeling diminished, is true humility.

Secondly, a humble heart acknowledges sin. It's hard to come before God with a humble heart and say, "My interests and time are most important. It's about me!" When I do, I am eating humble pie. There is nutritional value in eating humble pie—it will keep the soul shielded from those fiery darts.

Reflect: Peter counsels us on how to implement this process. First, read 1 Peter 5: 5–9 out loud. Then, reflect on how you can put this into practice.

1. *Humble yourself* by recognizing and then resisting all forms of pride.

2. *Cast all your anxiety onto God.* We need to ask God and others for help in order to grow. Sometimes the only thing standing in the way of great mind change is our fear that it is a sign of weakness to ask (which is pride).

3. *Be self-controlled.* We need to stop, think, and pray before rushing in or impulsively making key decisions.

4. *Be alert!* Our country has a *National Terror Alert Level* to disseminate information regarding the risk of terrorist acts. It is rated "low" to "severe." We institute a similar system. Anytime the "low" alert alarm sounds, we move into position. We don't wait until it hits severe.

5. *Resist Satan.* When attacked, say out loud, "Away from me Satan! In the name of Jesus Christ I command you to leave" (Matt. 4:10; Acts 16:18).

6. *Stand firm in the faith.* You are a brand new person inside and not the same anymore. A new life has begun! (2 Cor. 5:17)

A Grateful Mind and Heart

When you wake up in the morning, do you say, "Good morning, Lord," or, "Good Lord, it's morning!" Failure to be thankful, or to glorify and honor God, is a present-day problem. The Bible has long embraced gratitude as an indispensable virtue, but now there are scientific studies praising thankfulness and gratitude as an integral component of health, wholeness, and well-being.

The prize: a better functioning brain and heart and the peace of God! People who approach life with an attitude of gratitude are generally healthier, happier, and not depressed. It is now one of the treatment modalities for people with depression. It's harder for seeds of depression to take root in a grateful heart.

What about when things don't turn out, like disasters, accidents, abuse, job losses, or cancer? The Bible instructs us to "give thanks in *all* circumstances, for this is God's will for you in Christ Jesus" (1 Thess. 5:18). Stay with me. We learned God does not cause bad stuff to happen. He may allow it, but we have the assurance that in the midst of a trying circumstance, he is working in it. Nothing, even though it may have the earmarks of Satan all over it, can separate us from his love and mercy.

Sports legend and businessman Michael Jordan once said, "I've failed over and over and over again in my life. And that is why I succeed."[145] The failure rate in life is 100 percent. God actually prepares to bless us through our failures. Just look at the record of Abraham, Moses, David, Paul, and Peter to name five of many. They were no different than you and I. Each one ended up changing his world for God. Today, they are considered legends and successes.

God works by paradox. Success comes via failure, as life springs out of death. The only element in our lives that falls apart is that which has to go anyway. We eventually learn how to leave behind what God wants us to leave behind. It is our responsibility to accept God's perfect provision of grace and power because his power is made perfect in our weakness. God's provision empowers us against all enemies.

Reflect: Being thankful in a dire situation can only be done by faith. We can't do it in our own strength. Pray, "Father, I'm in a bad place right now. I don't want to be here, but you, in your love and wisdom allowed or chose it for me. I thank you for what you are about to do. Help me to believe this with my mind, my heart, and entire soul."

Thank You Lord!

I mentioned my "messenger of Satan" was when an interview with a high-profile ministry got bumped repeatedly. The interview eventually was released on CD. Holding that little piece of plastic, I was ecstatic. *Praise God! Thank you, Lord!* Then I listened to the interview. It was done well. But this organization did not mention my book or refer to it as a resource! I was hurt, disappointed, a bit bitter.

When I was a young girl, for my eighth birthday I asked for a new Barbie doll and the Barbie sports car. For months I envisioned me and Barbie driving everywhere together. The big day came. I couldn't tear the wrapping paper off fast enough. My mind was way ahead. *In a few moments, my hot new Barbie will be driving down the highway of our hallway in her new cool sports car! Where shall we go first, Barbie?*

Wait a minute... where's the car? All that's in this package is a new Barbie doll. I got gypped! That's how I felt when I listened to the interview. I took my feelings to God and confessed I was being ungrateful. Instead of thanking God for the Barbie doll, I was griping because I didn't get the car. It was a woe is me moment. Score: Satan!

The Bible says, "Be sure to fear the LORD and serve him faithfully with all your heart; consider what great things he has done for you" (1 Sam. 12:24). Think of all the blessings in your life. It's usually hard to be negative.

Luke tells the story about ten lepers who asked Jesus for healing. They were all cleansed. "One of them, when he saw he was healed, came back, praising God in a loud voice....Jesus said, "Rise and go; your faith has made you well" (Luke 17:15, 19).

Sadly, only one of the ten came back. The leper didn't thank God so he could get more. He just thanked God. I challenge you to change the cycle of thinking from: "What do I need?" to "Thank you Lord for what I have."

Give thanks for what God has done. Here are some suggestions:

1. *Everyday tell God five things you are thankful for.*

As hard as this is in tough times, we focus on what we have. One man was renowned for his cheerful endurance while going through a painful trial, "First, I look *within* me, then *without* me, afterwards *beneath* me, and last of all, *above* me."

He looked within and saw such guilt and unworthiness that whatever blessings balanced his afflictions, they were more than he deserved. He looked without and saw those who had far many more problems than himself. He looked beneath and saw the earth, into which his body would soon be lowered, and when all of life's trials would be over once and for all. He looked above and saw by faith his home in heaven, and this made the light affliction but for a moment, not worthy to be compared with the glory waiting to be revealed.

You *always* have at least one thing to be thankful for. This includes other people. Tell those other people what it is about them you are thankful for. Embrace God's little blessings: The air you breathe, your family, reliable transportation, groceries, hot water to shower with. You begin the process of cultivating a thankful spirit.

When was the last time you thanked God for your salvation or for delivering you from the domain of darkness and transferring you to the kingdom of light or thanked him for your health, intellectual ability, talents and gifts, instead of focusing on what you are not good at or don't have?

2. *Write a gratitude letter.*

"Thank you for participating in my life because ... " Pick three people—a relative, friend, and a person that influenced you. Not only will your life be more joyful—so will theirs! "Whatever you do, whether in word or deed, do it all in the name of the Lord Jesus, giving thanks to God the Father through him" (Col. 3:17).

3. *Praise others.*

Try to catch your kids, or employees, or spouse doing something right and praise them for it. There are countless reasons to praise our children. "Your drawing is incredible!" "Thank you for helping." Sam Walton, founder of Wal-Mart said, "Nothing else can quite substitute for a few well-chosen, well-timed, sincere word of praise. They're absolutely free, and worth a fortune."[146]

4. *Do something nice for someone secretly.* This is Christ in action.

Reflect: A mindset that says, "God's given me plenty" will strengthen emotionally and empower practically. Read Psalm 92:1–5. Begin by doing at least one of the four things mentioned to begin changing your mindset.

R.E.S.I.S.T. Recap

Recognize it is through grace that God renews your mind and brings you freedom to live a new life. He is also your power behind loving others—even the unlovable!

Embrace gratitude as an indispensable virtue. Begin to give thanks in *all* circumstances. Change the cycle of thinking from, "What do I need?" to "Thank you Lord for what I have."

Submit the pride in your heart and mind. Allow Jesus to shape you with humility. Your success comes from God.

Identify & Interrogate the state of your heart and mind today. Do you have a mind of humility? Humility will keep your soul shielded from those fiery darts.

Set your mind and heart on God. Like the man in the tombs, run toward Jesus, setting you entire soul on the redeemer. Every day fall down at his feet and accept his amazing grace and love.

Thank and Praise God! Every day look for new opportunities to praise and worship God; to serve and uplift others.

Kimberly Davidson

The Unmasked Life

Our ultimate hope is not perfection of character in this life, but in the perfection of character in eternity. John said, "we are already God's children, right now, and we can't even imagine what it is going to be like later on. But we do know this, that when he [*Jesus*] comes we will be like him" (1 John 3:2, TLB). The challenging process of being transformed into Christ's likeness will be over!

God never leaves anything incomplete. He has a plan for mankind: to remove the curse that came on this earth and restore eternal life. Jesus's work—the cross and the resurrection, took care of that. The battle we've been through, the one which is still going on, eventually comes to an end. God reveals the removal of the curse in the book of Revelation (22:2–3).

Revelation is not a book of cataclysmic predictions of doom and gloom, but a vision of Jesus and the abundant hope-filled life he wants for all his children. God finishes off evil, "The devil, who deceived them, was thrown into the lake of burning sulfur, where the beast and the false prophet had been thrown [*hell*]" (Rev. 20:10). So when Satan reminds you of your past, you remind him of his future!

Then another major event happens. A book is opened, which is the book of life where every believer's name is written (Rev. 20:12). *On that day we all will be accountable to God for what we did on this earth; also known as judgment day or retribution (2 Cor. 5:10;* Heb. *9:27). Retribution means you get something for what you do. Your account is settled.*

Many Christians think they will be ushered into heaven with no questions asked about their faithfulness on earth. Through Christ's payment on the cross, we have escaped eternal judgment (John 5:24); however, our actions will be judged. If God is to remain true to who he is, he must dispense justice and grace. Because God is absolutely just, we will be called to give an account of our actions. The Christian life gives tremendous freedom, but it also brings a pervasive sense of accountability to God. It also gives us a powerful reason to please God.

So what's left? The best part. God's final act of creation, "I am making everything new!" (Gen. 1:1, Rev. 21:5). He starts this creative move with a passed-away heaven and earth. Here comes a new heaven and a new earth—not to be confused with Eckhart Tolle's *A New Earth*. God will wipe away all tears from our eyes, and there shall be no more death, nor sorrow, nor crying, nor pain. All of that has gone forever (Rev. 21:4).

Then God reveals his grand plan of all time—relationship. "The dwelling of God is with men, and he will live with them" (Rev. 21:3). This is all God has ever wanted—to live among us, to interconnect, as our God and Father. What a family reunion! Nothing is more foundational to freedom and joy than understanding and feeling you are a child of God. No one else has ever been created to be and do what God has in mind for you.

We've all asked, "What am I here for? What is my destiny?" Only time with God will answer that. I can tell you that each Christian is called to be Jesus's representative. Singer Barry Manilow's classic, *Just One Voice*, says it well, "Just one voice, singing in the darkness, all it takes is one voice, singing so they hear what's on your mind, and when you look around you'll find there's more than one voice, singing in the darkness, joining with your one voice...hands are joined and fears unlocked, if only one voice would start it on its own, we need just one voice facing the unknown, and everyone will sing!"

We are not merely to avoid the world. "Preach the gospel everyday; if necessary, use words" (Francis of Assisi).[147] People are watching the way we act more than they are listening to what we say. Our challenge is to be an ambassador for Christ who lives by the truth. Jesus has done so very much for you. Don't stay silent. Take what you have learned and teach your loved ones. Look for opportunities to tell friends and family what great things the Lord has done.

The days ahead will be filled with opportunities intended

to entice you to invest your time and energy away from God. Never stop learning. The demon Screwtape told his protégé to keep knowledge out of the human's mind. The Bible says only fools hate knowledge (Prov. 1:22). Another reason, "Anyone who stops learning is old. Anyone who keeps learning stays young" (Henry Ford).[148]

Every day we will encounter new trials, temptations, and tests. But, today, you are living a brand new kind of life. Don't allow the enemy to crowd God's Word from your mind. "Do not be anxious about anything, [*anxiousness and worry are fiery darts from the devil*] but in everything, by prayer and petition, with thanksgiving, present your requests to God. And the peace of God, which transcends all understanding, will guard your hearts and your minds in Christ Jesus" (Phil. 4:6–7, *my emphasis*).

Mr. Keating in *Dead Poets Society* proclaimed, "Carpe diem. Seize the day, boys [*ladies*]. Make your lives extraordinary!"

Appendix

The Bible: The Power of God's Word and Thoughts

In the Old Testament, the finger of God wrote the Ten Commandments on stone tablets and later he inscribed a message on the walls of Belshazzar's palace. In the New Testament, the finger of Jesus wrote in the dirt. Today we have God's handwriting in the Holy Bible. The Bible (the word *Bible* means book), is also referred to as *Scripture* or the *Word of God*. All Scripture is inspired by God and each word *is* God's holy Word (2 Tim. 3:16). It is our authority, power, and source of guidance for our faith and lives.

The Word of God, the Bible, is inerrant—it does not make a mistake; is infallible—it is flawless; and is inspired by God himself. It is truth. Known as revelation, God self-discloses himself to mankind because we were created to know God. It is his powerful and meaningful self-expression. Every time I open my Bible, God is speaking to me personally!

Four Reasons for Reading the Bible:

1. It is the Christian's authority and standard for living. The Bible's power rests upon the fact that it is reliable and the perfect Word of God.

2. The Bible speaks to us individually. Only when we take the Word of God into our minds and hearts do we come to know the truth and begin to break down toxic thinking. It literally has the capacity to transform our heart and

mind and body—our attitudes and actions into the image of Christ.

3. The Bible is not merely a source of helpful suggestions, preventative warnings, or inspirational thoughts; it is life itself. It speaks to our day because it speaks to our soul—our inner nature.

4. It enables the reader to understand the Christian faith. The death of Jesus was a divine plan. God will save humanity and Israel!

The Bible consists of two parts: the Old Testament, which has been called the Hebrew Scriptures, and later writings known as the New Testament. The Old Testament is the collection of thirty-nine books written prior to the life of Jesus. It is the story of the covenant of God with Israel and the prophetic anticipation of Jesus's coming to redeem the people of God.

The New Testament is a collection of twenty-seven books, of three different genres of Christian literature: The Gospels, which relate the life and teachings of Jesus; the letters of the Apostle Paul and other disciples to the early church called the Acts of the Apostles and the Epistles; and the Book of Revelation, an Apocalypse. The New Testament is fulfilled in the coming of Jesus. He is the central figure.

Human beings cannot reach up to study God, and even if they could, would not understand him. Through the Holy Spirit, God revealed what he wanted to reveal of himself through the use of human beings and human language (2 Pet. 1:20–21).

Through the Bible a personal God presents himself to us. We need his Word in order to think his thoughts and know the whole truth, as much as humanly possible. We also need it to do its corrective work and allow it to protect us from the world's wisdom—from falsehoods. I challenge you to begin to look at the Bible differently.

Endnotes

1 Justsell.com, February 16, 2009

2 Caroline Leaf, *Who Switched Off My Brain*, Backmatter, Switch On Your Brain Organisation Pty (Ltd.), 2007

3 JustSell.com, April 9, 2009

4 Caroline Leaf, *Who Switched Off My Brain*, 113-114, Switch On Your Brain Organisation Pty (Ltd.), 2007

5 Ibid, 8, 113-114, 94

6 David Jeremiah, *Turning Points*, February 23, 2009

7 Just sell.com, July 9, 2008

8 Anne Moir, *Brain Sex: The Real Difference Between Men and Women*, 33-37, New York: Dell Publishing, 1991

9 Daniel G. Amen, M.D., "Healing the Hardware of the Soul," http://www.amenclinic.com/bp/articles.php?articleID=20

10 *Brain In the News*, "Child Abuse 'Impacts Stress Gene,'" March, 2009

11 http://www.youmeworks.com/sendablessing.html; Accessed August 16, 2008

12 John Townsend, *Who's Pushing Your Buttons*, 22, Nashville: Integrity Publishers, 2004

13 Neil Anderson, *The Bondage Breaker*, 69, 72, Eugene: Harvest House, 2000, 2nd Rev.

14 Soul Care, *New Every Morning*, September 4, 2008

15 Ibid, March 10, 2009

16 Archibald Hart, "Lovers of Pleasures," *Christian Counseling Today*, 13, Vol. 16 No. 2, 2009

17   C.S. Lewis, *The Screwtape Letters*, 39-40, New York: The Macmillan Company, 1960

18   See: Lev. 19:26, 31; 20:6; Deut. 18:9-13; Acts 19:18-20

19   Cornelius Plantinga, Jr., *Not the Way It's Supposed to Be*, 95, Grand Rapids: William B. Eerdmans, 1995

20   Dan Boone, *Answers for Chicken Little*, 54, Kansas City: Beacon Hill Press, 2005

21   Neil Anderson, *Victory Over Darkness*, 103, Ventura: Regal Books, 1990

22   Robert S. McGee, *The Search for Freedom*, 26, Ann Arbor: Vine Books, 1995

23   Health.com, 2009

24   Les Carter, "Anti-Growth Trait," e-newsletter February, 2009; www.drlescarter.com

25   *Science*, October 10th issue, http://mentalhealth.about.com/b/2003/10/16/rejection-feels-like-pain-to-the-brain.htm

26   Walt Larimore, M.D., *God's Design for the Highly Healthy Teen*, 250, Grand Rapids: Zondervan, 2005

27   Ibid, 22-23

28   Charles Colson and Harold Fickett, Focus On The Family, "It's Not My Fault," September 2008

29   Mary Pipher, PhD, *Reviving Ophelia*, 25, New York: Ballantine Books, 1994

30   Soul Care *New Every Morning*, April 7, 2009

31   Carrington Steele, *Don't Drink the Kool-Aid*, 1, © 2008 Carrington Steele

32   Francis Brown, S.R. Driver and Charles Briggs, *Hebrew and English Lexicon of the Old Testament*, 966, New York: Oxford University Press, 1955

33   http://en.wikipedia.org/wiki/Lucifer; Accessed July 17, 2008

34   C.S. Lewis, *Mere Christianity*, 53, 1952; 1980

35   The Internet Movie Database: http://www.imdb.com/
      title/tt0052520/quotes; accessed December 24, 200

36   Paul Tripp, *War of Words*, 25, Phillips-
      burg: P&R Publishing, 2000

37   David Jeremiah, *Turning Points*, July 3, 2008

38   John Owen, *Communication with God*, 13, ed. R.J.K.Law,
      Edinburgh Scotland: The Banner of Truth Trust, 1991

39   David Jeremiah, *Turning Points*, March 25, 2009

40   JustSell.com, January 30, 2009

41   Caroline Leaf, *Who Switched Off My Brain*, 19-20,
      Switch On Your Brain Organisation Pty (Ltd.), 2007

42   http://www.quotedb.com/categories/pride/rating

43   David Jeremiah, *Turning Points*, February 14, 2009

44   Donald Stuss, Neuroscientist, Baycrest's Rotman
      Research Institute: *Brain In The News*, "It's Never
      Too Late to grow Your Brain," December 2008

45   Pat O'Connor *Friendships Between Women*,
      17, New York: Guilford Press, 1992

46   www.nccam.nih.gov; AARP, Jan. & Feb.
      2009, "Health Report," 34

47   M. Scott Peck, M.D, *People of the Lie*, 60,
      New York: Simon and Schuster, 1983

48   Daniel G. Amen, M.D., *Change Your Brain, Change Your
      Life*, 44, 47, New York: Three Rivers Press, 1998

49   Ibid, 3

50   Daniel G. Amen, M.D., *Healing the Hardware of
      the Soul*, 6, New York: The Free Press, 2002

51   Dan Allender, *The Wounded Heart*, 101, 103,
      Colorado Springs: NavPress, 1990

52   Marge Engleman, *Your Amazing Brain and How It
      Works*, 9, Verona: Attainment Company, 2008

53   http://www.healthylivingnyc.com/article/128; accessed January 29, 2008

54   Soul Care, *New Every Morning,* November 6, 2008

55   Wikipedia: http://en.wikipedia.org/wiki/Mind

56   Sharon Begley, John Carey, and Ray Sawhill, 40, "How the Brain Works," *Newsweek* 7 February 7, 1983.

57   Daniel G. Amen, M.D., "Healing the Hardware of the Soul," http://www.amenclinic.com/bp/articles.php?articleID=20

58   http://findarticles.com/p/articles/mi_qn4179/is_20000414/ai_n11744685; Accessed August 12, 2008

59   Soul Care: New Every Morning, March 27, 2009

60   Daniel G. Amen, M.D., *Healing the Hardware of the Soul,* 32-33, New York: The Free Press, 2002

61   Ibid, 34, 37

62   Ibid, 62, 65-66, 74

63   Ibid, 58

64   *Brain in the News,* "Study Links Depression to Thinning of Brain's Cortex," April 2009, (The New York Times, March, 2009, Section A, 17)

65   Daniel G. Amen, M.D., *Change Your Brain, Change Your Life,* 6-7, New York: Three Rivers Press, 1998

66   Walt Larimore, M.D., *God's Design for the Highly Healthy Teen,* 205, Grand Rapids: Zondervan, 2005

67   Daniel G. Amen, M.D. *Making a Good Brain Great,* 152, New York: Three Rivers Press, 2005

68   Caroline Leaf, *Who Switched Off My Brain,* 4, 8, 125, Switch On Your Brain Organisation Pty (Ltd.), 2007

69   John Ortberg, *God Is Closer Than You Think,* Grand Rapids: Zondervan, 2005

70   Walt Larimore, M.D., *God's Design for the Highly Healthy Teen,* 199, Grand Rapids: Zondervan, 2005

71   The Way of the Master Evidence Bible, 1952, Orlando: Bridge-Logos, 2003

72   Patsy Clairmont, *I Second that Emotion,* 11, Nashville: Thomas Nelson, 2008

73   Sharon A. Hersh, *Mom, I Hate My Life!* 40, Colorado Springs: Shaw Books, 2004

74   Dan Allender and Trempter Longman III, *The Cry of the Soul,* 26, Colorado Springs: NavPress, 1994

75   http://en.wikipedia.org/wiki/Temptation; accessed December 1, 2007

76   http://thinkexist.com/quotation/i_generally_avoid_temptation_unless_i_can-t/168998.html; accessed December 1, 2007

77   Ibid, April 14, 2008

78   JustSell.com; December 4, 2008

79   Vance Havner, *Pleasant Paths,* 74, Grand Rapids: Baker Book House, 1945

80   Charles Haddon Spurgeon, *Spurgeon's Sermons, Vol. 1,* 126-127, Grand Rapids: Baker Book House, 1983

81   Cheryl Forbes, *Imagination,* Quoted in: David Needham, *Birthright: Christian, Do You Know Who You Are?,* 184-185, Sisters: Multonomah Publishers, 1999

82   Tim Hartford, "How to Save Smarter," *Parade,* 10, May 10, 2009

83   Caroline Leaf, *Who Switched Off My Brain,* 111-112, Switch On Your Brain Organisation Pty (Ltd.), 2007

84   Ibid, 114-115

85   Ibid.

86   David Jeremiah, *Turning Points,* June 1, 2009

87   AACC, *Christian Counseling Connection,* "For The Record: The Foster Report," USA Today: 1/10/06, 2007/Issue 2

88   A. W. Tozer, *Tozer Topical Reader,* comp. Ron Eggert, 2.185, Camp Hill: Christian Publications, 1998

89   Larry Crabb, *Christian Counseling Today,* "Perfectionism: Good or Bad?," 58, Vol. 16 No. 2, 2009

90   Charles Colson and Harold Fickett, Focus On The Family, "It's Not My Fault," September 2008

91   JustSell.com, May 26, 2008

92   John MacArthur, *The Truth War*, xx-xxi, Nashville: Thomas-Nelson, 2008

93   Jim Andrews, Polishing God's Monuments, 139-140, Wapwallopen: Shepherd Press, 2007

94   Warren Wiersbe, *The Strategy of Satan*, 47, Wheaton: Tyndale, 1979

95   JustSell.com; December 17, 2008

96   http://www.lyricsfreak.com/g/garth+brooks/unanswered+prayers_20058116.html; Accessed April 14, 2008

97   Robert W. Kelleman, *Beyond the Suffering: Embracing the Legacy of African-American Soul Care and Spiritual Direction*, 214-215, Grand Rapids: Baker Books, 2007

98   Soul Care New Every Morning, January 28, 2009

99   Paul Brand and Philip Yancey, *In His Image,* 33, Grand Rapids: Zondervan, 1987

100   Gerry Breshears, Western Seminary, THS 502, Portland, Oregon

101   SoulCare New Every Morning, April 1, 2009

102   Daniel G. Amen, M.D., *Change Your Brain, Change Your Life,* 299, New York: Three Rivers Press, 1998

103   CNN.com, *Mother Teresa's Letters Reveal Doubts*, September 7, 2001, accessed February 16, 2008

104   Les Cater, "The Deepest Problem," www.drlescarter.com; received: April 1, 2008

105   Lewis Smedes, *Shame and Grace: Healing the Shame We Don't Deserve*, 116, San Francisco: Harper Collins, 1993

106   Gary McIntosh and Samuel Rima, Sr., *Overcoming the Dark Side of Leadership*, 13, 22-23, Grand Rapids: Baker Books, 1997

107 C.S. Lewis, *The Screwtape Letters,* 20-21, New York: The Macmillan Company, 1960

108 Reported by Jeffrey Zaslow, "Straight Talk," *USA Weekend,* 18, February 7-9, 1997

109 Gary McIntosh and Samuel Rima, Sr., *Overcoming the Dark Side of Leadership,* 156-157, Grand Rapids: Baker Books, 1997

110 Miles J. Stanford, *The Complete Green Letters,* 41, Grand Rapids: Zondervan, 1983

111 Dwight L. Moody Quotes: http://thinkexist.com/quotes/dwight_l._moody/3.html; accessed June 2, 2008

112 Sinclair B. Ferguson, *John Owen on the Christian Life,* 125, Edinburgh, Scotland: The Banner Truth Trust, 1987

113 Daniel G. Amen, M.D. *Making a Good Brain Great,* 8, New York: Three Rivers Press, 2005

114 Ibid, 13-14

115 Ibid, 15

116 Daniel G. Amen, M.D., *Change Your Brain, Change Your Life,* 56, New York: Three Rivers Press, 1998

117 David Jeremiah, *Turning Points,* August 14, 2008

118 Archibald Hart, "Lovers of Pleasures," *Christian Counseling Today,* 13, Vol. 16 No. 2, 2009

119 Pete A. Sanders, Jr., *Access Your Brain's Joy Center: The Free Soul Method,* 3, Sedona: Free Soul, 1996

120 Jerry Bridges, *Respectable Sins,* 41, Colorado Springs: NavPress, 2007

121 See Rom. 15:16; 1 Cor. 6:11, 2 Cor. 3:18, 1 John 3:2

122 Daniel G. Amen, M.D., *Change Your Brain, Change Your Life,* 56, New York: Three Rivers Press, 1998

123 Michael Dye and Patricia Fancher, "Relapse and the Brain," http://www.nacronline.com/dox/library/sub_relapse.shtml; Accessed May 6, 2008

124 Pete A. Sanders, Jr., *Access Your Brain's Joy Center: The Free Soul Method*, 3, Sedona: Free Soul, 1996

125 Michael Dye and Patricia Fancher, "Relapse and the Brain," http://www.nacronline.com/dox/library/sub_relapse.shtml; Accessed May 6, 2008

126 http://itc.conversationsnetwork.org/shows/detail733.html

127 Daniel Amen, M.D, *Using Brain Imaging in Understanding and Treating Addictions*, American Association of Christian Counselors, "No Greater Love," September, 2007; http://amenclinics.com/ac/waystohelp.php?refWays=marital

128 Daniel G. Amen, M.D. *Making a Good Brain Great*, 63, New York: Three Rivers Press, 2005

129 Jordan Rubin, "The Genesis of Our Downfall," *Enjoying Everyday Life*, 30, March/April 2009

130 Barbara Anan Kogan, "You Think What You Eat," May/June *Vibrant Life*, Hagerstown, MD, 2008

131 Ibid

132 Daniel G. Amen, M.D., *Change Your Brain, Change Your Life*, 27-28, New York: Three Rivers Press, 1998

133 Healthcom, "Special Report," May 2009

134 Micheal R. Lyles, M.D., "Healthy Weight Management Strategies," *Christian Counseling Today*, 13, Vol. 16 No. 2, 2009

135 Daniel J. DeNoon, *WebMD Health News*, "Lack of Sleep Takes Toll on Brain Power," Feb. 9, 2000

136 Andrew Purves, *Pastoral Theology in the Classic Tradition*,' Gregory of Nazianzus, Oration 2.71, :In defense of His Flight to Pontus," 9, Louisville: Westminster John Knox Press, 2001

137 Roger Walsh, *Essential Spirituality*, 200, John Wiley & Sons, 2000

138 David Jeremiah, *Turning Points*, May 9, 2009

139 Donald S. Whitney, *Spiritual Disciplines for the Christian Life*, 152, Colorado Springs: NavPress, 1991

140   Jerry Bridges, *Respectable Sins,*123, Colo-
      rado Springs: NavPress, 2007

141   Patsy Clairmont, *I Second that Emotion,*
      24, Nashville: Thomas Nelson, 2008

142   Ibid, March 17, 2009

143   Soul Care New Every Morning, August 20, 2008

144   Ibid, September 5, 2008

145   Justsell.com, March 28, 2008

146   Ibid, November 14, 2008

147   David Jeremiah, *Turning Points*, September 4, 2008

148   Justsell.com, September 30, 2008